The Book of Love

A Schizophrenic's Discoveries from a Metaphysical, Spiritual Awakening

by Eddie Faggioli

Self-Published by Eddie Faggioli on Create Space,
www.Amazon.com
Please direct questions to Eddie Faggioli:
Eddie.Faggioli@Yahoo.com

Editing: Dr. Graves, Paul Weisser, and E.M. Levy
Production: Eddie Faggioli
Type design: Eddie Faggioli
Cover design: Eddie Faggioli
Cover art: Pamela Fessel (On Facebook under, Pamela Fessel's Artwork)

Library of Congress Catalog-in-Publication Data
Faggioli, Eddie

The Book of Love: A Schizophrenic's Discoveries from a Metaphysical, Spiritual Awakening / Eddie Faggioli
Book: 1 Edition: 1.0
ISBN-13: 978-1727285925
Genre: Memoir

Printed in the United States of America

Table of Contents

Disclaimers

This book is not meant to diagnose, cure, or treat any illness, directly or indirectly. It is only for your well-being, as we assume no responsibility for your actions.

If after reading this book, you choose to take part in having a spiritual experience such as channeling, we forwarn you that any channeling can expose you to both the light and the darkness. Therefore we assume no responsibility for your spiritual experiences.

There is also adult language in this book, so reader discretion is advised.

This book does not, directly or indirectly reflect the views of any businesses mentioned in it. The trademarks of these businesses belong to their respective companies.

Acknowledgments

I would like to pay heartfelt honor to those individuals who helped to put this book together: to God and the Divine; to psychic Leo for giving me friendly insight without judgment; to Savannah for all her loving help—my love for you is as deep as the ocean; to Dr. Graves for his amazing legal support; to Pam for the artwork; to Travis Walker for his amazing assistance; to Paul Weisser for his expertise; to the hacker who altered this book and taught me about privacy; and to E. M. Levy for rescuing this project. You have all set me up for the future in respective ways for which I can't give enough thanks. Honestly, where would I be without you?

To the dreamer within you, reader, may you receive everything your heart and soul desire.

To open-minded and "seeking" individuals, I hope this book leaves you utterly fascinated.

Preface

If you haven't knowingly come into contact with a schizophrenic, you should be aware that 51 million people are schizophrenic—or 1.1 percent of the world's population.[1] That means that roughly one in every hundred people will have the disease at some point in their lifetime. Therefore, you have probably come into contact with a schizophrenic at some time in your life.

What has shaped your view of schizophrenics? The media has publicized the few schizophrenics who have harmed other people but have not portrayed a greater picture. According to *schizophrenia.com*, schizophrenics are "linked" by the media for having both a mental illness and committing a crime, but they are mostly nonviolent, and when they are violent, it is mostly toward themselves. A survey in 2006 found that 60 percent of Americans think that people with schizophrenia are likely to act violently toward someone else, and 32 percent think that people who

---

[1]*Schizophrenia.com/szfacts.htm.*

have major depression will harm others.[2] Actually, substance abuse is more likely to be a contributing factor in violent crime than one's mental health.

Schizophrenia.com explains that schizophrenics are more likely to withdraw from the public and seek to be left alone. If they commit a crime and receive a jail sentence, it is more likely to be for misdemeanors such as trespassing than for violence. Individuals with "severe" psychiatric disorders, such as schizophrenics, who do not take their medication are 2.7 times more likely to be the victim of a violent crime (such as assault, rape, or mugging) than the average person.[3]

As I was writing this book, a character you will later read about, whom I call Savannah, brought something interesting to my attention.

"Remember when everyone first found out about AIDS?" she said. "No one wanted to live with an AIDS patient. Then research discovered that it would take a gallon of saliva to transfer AIDS orally, and it was also not likely to be spread via contact with a toothbrush or a

---

[2]*Health.harvard.edu/newsletter_article/mental-illness-and-violence/.*
[3]*Mentalillnesspolicy.org/consequences/victimization.html/.*

bathtub. People were relieved by those facts, and AIDS patients became more acceptable to live among."

Savannah and I believe that the same thing is true of schizophrenia. Not much is known about it right now, but the research usually makes the disease more acceptable than the stigma associated with it.

As a schizophrenic myself, I feel that we are usually misunderstood. Many schizophrenics have what are classified as "hallucinations" and "delusions," which make us sound scary or incredibly abnormal. Some schizophrenics who reach this level of "insanity" don't always recover enough to articulate what happened to them, which can be difficult to put into words.

After I recovered enough from my own schizophrenia, with the help of therapy and medications, I experienced a different side of spirituality than many other non-psychics' experience. My aim in writing this book is to present my own experiences, without trying to be right or wrong. In other words, I am not arguing any viewpoint; by keeping a student-of-God perspective, without pushing any spiritual beliefs or views onto others, I am simply saying what happened. This is just a spiritual journey and an individual quest to find my own road to truth. Therefore, if anything I say doesn't agree with you, please don't be offended.

Where I am spiritually in the present moment is not necessarily where I will be in the future, since I am always learning. I believe that I am just driving on God's road, not knowing where I'll end up. You, of course, are free to believe whatever resonates with your own belief system. I just want to describe my personal experiences in the hope that others will find them interesting, thoughtful, or spiritually helpful.

By the same token, I also don't want others to push their beliefs on me. This is just a memoir of my journeys. I believe it's worth communicating things in order to create a greater future. Even in a conflict, each point of view contains some level of truth, regardless of how "crazy" it may sound at first.

Therefore, I ask that you withhold judging me. A method spiritual people apply to withhold judgment is to not associate something (me) with a value, such as "good" or "bad." Doing this will decrease the dramatic effect of my story, as you will be merely observing what happened, if you choose to do so.

Nonetheless, I hope the byproduct of this book will be to create a higher path for our work and a more therapeutic environment for individuals with schizophrenia, one that is conducive to and supports spiritual awakening.

However, after being described as psychotic by the mental-health industry, I do hope to shape the perceptions of clinicians around the world and to convey to them the idea that what schizophrenics experience is probably less "delusional" than it appears from the outside. Although I am not a physician and don't have a scientific or medical degree, I do believe I have recovered enough from schizophrenia to have insights into my personal experiences and perceptions. To be precise, clinicians attempt to analyze schizophrenia from the outside in, whereas I attempt to describe my experience from the inside out.

I do hope we will begin to realize that we are all beautifully unique, and none of us should ever be spoken to with distain or mistreated for our lower experiences, as love is the glue that holds us together.

One theme I would like to continuously come back to in my books and music is that we're all connected and that love is the highest form of truth. Therefore, what we do to others we do to ourselves, and what we do to ourselves we do to others.

For example, to cause suffering to another is to cause suffering to yourself, and to cause suffering to yourself will cause suffering to those who watch you do it. Conversely, to cause great help to others is to create great feelings within, and to cause great feelings within is to create greatness outside of yourself, as you will observe in the chapter on the law of attraction.

Because this book was written over a period of years, a spiritual reader may notice how my thoughtforms evolved from using judgmental words to higher states of love. In other words, my writing progresses with my vibration, as I grow spiritually over the course of the book.

I have also tried to state a higher truth here about the people I have described, including the "bad" with the "good," or as I say the "lower" information with the "higher." As a result, there are technically no good guys or bad guys. If you look for the bad guys, you may find yourself first disliking and then loving them; that will just be a result of my attempt to shape a fuller viewpoint about that character.

My purpose is to describe spiritual experiences that many unawakened people may view as impossibilities. Anyone who feels that way probably hasn't gotten to know spirituality at a deep psychic level yet. Therefore, in an attempt to preserve my integrity, I frequently cite spiritual and academic research to back up my points with non-schizophrenics' spiritual experiences. I believe that although my journey shares some slight differences, it has many commonalities to the spiritual experiences of non-schizophrenics as well.

Quite a few perfectly sane individuals have become spiritually evolved but don't speak about their spiritual experiences because they don't want to risk being judged, medicated, or institutionalized. In short, if you are awakened, you may find that we all can be a little bit schizophrenic in some ways. So, I have attempted here to structure a more accurate viewpoint on schizophrenia, based on my own real-life experiences.

In the following pages, I often refer to the "Divine," which means loving, heavenly beings in general, such as angels, guides, and ascended masters. None of the characters in this book worshiped the spirits, or beings that came through our psychic encounters, other than God.

I am a DJ by profession and have actually DJ'd this book, accompanying the text with songs. For the full experience, I encourage you to listen to the songs before reading the accompanying text each time, so the music doesn't interfere with your reading experience. The music I have prompted the reader to play, as artistic expressions of my story, are found in parentheses.

If you have ever felt that you were not good enough for other people, or were even cast out by them, I hope this book demonstrates that you can inspire others when you take an active role in your own growth and empowerment. We all have God and the power of God deep within our souls when we find the Christ-Self.

Before my journey as a schizophrenic, I was just an everyday person. Like you, I found that life at times was not easy. As the stress of my life came to a peak, I encountered a major obstacle that took me on two separate occasions to insanity and back. During the journey, I was brought to my knees with suffering that caused me to sincerely seek the wisdom of happiness. Through that wisdom, I learned secrets of the universe that returned me to a sane balance I never dreamed could happen. That is where my story begins.

In the Beginning

In 2006, I decided to contact one of my fellow graduates from trade college to see if he needed a carpenter. To my surprise, he was doing so well that he offered me carpentry work for $40 per hour. We worked together in the wealthy suburbs of King of Prussia and west Philadelphia. He and his superiors were impressed with my finish carpentry skills, but my state of mind began to show signs of a decline.

For some reason, I couldn't do regular things that most other tradesmen found easy. For example, I couldn't find job sites I had been to before, I had trouble conceptualizing the stages of construction and performing essential functions, and I couldn't understand why. This mental handicap crept in quickly, and before I knew it, I was experiencing things I didn't realize were out of the ordinary.

One morning, as I awoke from a terrible rest, the news reporter on the TV set was speaking directly to me.

"Eddie," he said, "when you drive east today, you need

to take these roads to avoid traffic."

When I started my car, a little later, the radio personalities were picking up where the news reporter left off.

"Eddie," one of them said, "you have become famous, and today you are going to start filming your movie . . . As you head east, you're going straight to Philadelphia, where the staging and cameras are already set up."

I was hypnotized. In this state of mind, I couldn't stop myself from listening to them or from doing what they said.

"Eddie," another one said, "it's time to do some stunt driving."

I began driving the wrong way down a highway. Cars raced out of my path as I drove down an "on" ramp to exit. As I entered Philadelphia, the city was remarkably empty. No one seemed to notice me driving the wrong way down one-way streets.

I took my work truck into a baseball field and cut a series of liberating donuts on the well-manicured grass. The engine was revving like a sports car. On my way out, I ran over a sign and dashed down the sidewalk. I squinted to try and make sense of what I was seeing, which led to me crashing into a large metal barrier, which prevented me from potentially crashing into a gas station.

As I got out of my wrecked truck, I decided to make this scene a little more bad-ass by getting a fresh new haircut at a barbershop nearby. In the end, I tipped the barber at least $20 and walked back to find that my truck was on the back of a tow truck.

A police officer who was looking down as he filled out his paperwork said to me in an almost casual tone, “Is this your truck?”

“Yeah,” I said.

“Then, you’re under arrest for a DUI.”

As he walked me back to the paddy wagon, someone drove by and yelled, “That’s the guy who was driving the wrong way down the highway!”

The officer continued to fill out paperwork for another ten minutes when I suddenly realized that this was becoming a drinking scene. So I decided to fall over inside the paddy wagon in a drunken stupor.

A moment later, the officer opened the back door of the paddy wagon and said sarcastically, “Are those cuffs too tight?" After loosening them and then tightening them as painfully as they were before, he said, "Usually, people sober up after being arrested."

I said, "I chugged the bottle right before I crashed."

The officer couldn't take any more of my nonsense, and brought me straight to the station's jail, where I was given a blood test and released three hours later.

After wandering around the streets for a while, I went into a huge Asian market to get a bite to eat. All this time, I felt like I was in a movie. Finally, it dawned on me that I should try to recover my wrecked, impounded truck, which in Philadelphia is difficult for *anyone* to do. So I wandered from building to building until nightfall.

As I was walking down the shoulder of a highway, my mother called me on my cell phone from Florida.

"Eddie, are you okay?"

"Yeah."

"Where are you?"

"I'm walking down the side of a highway."

"You can't do that," she replied simply. "Hold on." Then she hung up but called right back. "Eddie," she said, "I dispatched a police officer to your location."

Is she Superwoman?

Soon after she said that, I noticed a car creeping up behind me on the shoulder of the highway.

Am I going to the station again? Am I under arrest?

The police officer gently explained that he was going to drop me off at a train station, and clearly told me which stop I was supposed to get off. Then he reached into his pocket and gave me some of his own money for the fare.

What a caring police officer.

On the train, which felt breezy and calm, there were people behind me in formal business attire. I wondered if they were talking about me, so I would periodically turn to see. After the third time, they were huddled together, and I began to grow paranoid.

What are they going to do to me?

I got off the train at the next stop, which happened to be my home station, but as I approached the end of the parking lot, I couldn't understand why I could hear them laughing at me.

As soon as I reached the street, my uncle arrived in his Jeep to pick me up. I tried to speak to him but couldn't. The mental handicap of my condition was slowing my brain down to nothing. In fact, it became empty and thoughtless.

As the evening rain pattered down on the Jeep's rooftop, my uncle said, very casually, "I'm going to take you to this place . . . These people are just going to talk to you. They're going to ask you some questions and talk a little bit."

(At this point in the story, play Pink Floyd's "Time.")

Soon we were approaching the creepiest building I've ever seen. It gave me a horrible feeling in the pit of my stomach. To get to it, we had to go down an uncomfortably slow winding road.

I wonder what happens to people in there.

When we got inside, two large muscular men escorted my uncle into a small meeting room to the side, where they spoke together quietly. As he spoke, they appeared to be very sympathetic.

Everything seemed so surreal to me. Once again, I felt like I was living in a movie and began wandering around with nothing to do. To make the film more interesting, I lay down on a gurney, which is where the two men found me.

The first thing one of the men said was, "We're not going to have sex with you. We don't do that here."

Huh? . . . Sex? What are they talking about?

They hurried as they guided me through three sets of locked doors.

"We're going to take good care of you here," one of them said.

The next day, they attempted to play soothing music to people who looked like they were going insane from it. One guy got so distraught that he shoved a Bible at me and said, "Read it!"

I looked at him and took the Bible because I sensed that he would have beaten me to a pulp if I didn't. As I read the verses intently in my room, I could hear him yelling with reckless abandon, "The rapture is coming! The rapture is coming!"

Trying to quiet him down, the counselors said, "Shhh, there are other people living here. You don't want to disturb them."

A little later, I saw the hottest nurse I had ever seen in my life. I must have rubbed my eyes as if I were waking up slowly from a dream.

"What are you doing later?" I asked. "Maybe we could have some drinks."

She scowled at me as if she had been approached like this a hundred times before, and then just walked away.

I spent many days in that place, not knowing where I was or why I was there.

In my mental state, I figured that the only organization that could have the technology to create "hallucinations" and read my mind was the CIA. I was in a building being run by the CIA. The very caring psychiatrist kept giving me low doses of medication and asking if I were getting better. I didn't know any different, so I said, "Yeah."

In about two weeks, I was out again, back at my apartment.

Under medicated, I went insane in my efficiency, the demons were all over me and wouldn't leave me alone for even half a second. I found myself listening to Marilyn Manson and breaking windows in my apartment from the madness the demons were creating in my head.

The next day, I told my brother, Michael, who was a psychology major and lived right down the street, what I had done.

"You can't just throw a chair through your window," he said, laughing.

When he came to my apartment the next day, accompanied by the police, they found my front door wide open. The police immediately drew their guns and cautiously went inside, which they found empty, since I was out helplessly wandering the streets again.

The next morning, I awoke to a knock on my door. When I opened it, two huge men gently talked to me about my throwing a chair through the window, and then asked me to pack a bag and come with them. I was so terrified that I packed only a pair of underpants in a small bag and left with the men.

This time, because I admitted myself, I was brought to a different section of the hospital, which seemed to me like a hole in the wall. Located in the projects, it was equipped with broken furniture and blocked windows that didn't allow you to see fully outside. In other words, it felt like a jail.

My family was terrified when they realized that I had the same illness that had caused my father to commit suicide when I was eight. My mother was panicked, and when she spoke to my doctor every night, she kept telling him how poorly I was doing. The doctor then upped my meds so much that I was sure I was dying from a heart attack. I allowed him to do that, thinking that if I died, my family could sue the hospital.

Obviously, my family would rather have had me around than sue the hospital, but my distorted logic kept me from sticking up for myself. The problem with asserting yourself in a mental hospital is that it can postpone your release date if the doctors consider it resistance to treatment.

As I walked down the hallway in the old-fashioned clothing that had been donated to the hospital, the lights started flashing on and off. Suddenly, my soul lifted up out of my body, and I looked down at myself walking.

Am I actually dying? Are the lights actually flashing, or is it all in my head?

It felt so peaceful as it happened, like being in a state of meditation. The building seemed to quiet down during the experience.

At this rate, the medication (Seroquel) had me so high that I thought they were giving me straight marijuana.

When I sat down to eat dinner in the cafeteria, the boom box in the background was playing "We Are the Champions" by Queen. All the patients joined in as we spontaneously sang our hearts out. I got so carried away that I knocked over my drink and ran out of the cafeteria because I thought I was going to get in trouble.

During visiting hours, one of my sisters, Larissa, came to visit from Florida, along with Michael, but mostly they just spoke to each other.

"Why am I here?" I asked.

Michael said, "You have schizophrenia. You have to listen to the doctors to get better."

In my paranoid state, Michael was the only person I trusted to give me accurate information about my mental state. An angel in disguise, he was, in fact, the sole reason for my initial progress.

My caseworker was the second hottest girl I had ever seen.

Where did they hire these girls from? I'm going to behave this time.

Holding back tears, she explained to me that my illness was like the one the guy had in the movie *A Beautiful*

Mind.

“Where are the cameras, Eddie?” she asked sadly. “Don’t you see? This is all in your head.”

A New Life

When I was released from the hospital, again after two weeks, the Italian side of my family wanted to help me out and gave me work in the family demolition business. My medication fogged my mind, but I was still able to work hard. On the way home, however, the huge cutoff saw in the back of the company truck flew out as I was pulling off the highway. Unfortunately, I had forgotten to close the truck's gate.

As the saw, which is used to cut concrete, slid across traffic, it got lodged under an SUV, and sparks flew down on the highway as the saw literally disintegrated into nothing. Since I was so heavily medicated, I had no chance to react. That was the beginning of my realization that I was no longer the man I once was.

My uncle didn't want to leave me alone in the apartment I had lost my mind in, so he told me I could stay at his small house if I painted the bedroom. I painted the room a beautiful shade of bluish gray and felt so peaceful in my new "retreat." However, when I went to the leasing office to get my security deposit back, breaking my lease wasn't easy.

The manager of my apartment in King of Prussia didn't seem to regard a stay in a mental hospital as an excuse for moving out of my lease early. Fortunately, a large law firm in Philadelphia helped me when no one else would. The manager gave me my deposit back, but only because that was cheaper than paying a lawyer to fight the case in court.

I received a letter in the mail from my doctor, a signed document stating that I was "permanently disabled" and a lifetime candidate for Social Security.

Was I seriously permanently disabled? I hadn't come to my own conclusion. *How does the doctor define a disability?*

In 2007, I calculated that the absolute minimum I would need to live in Pennsylvania was $1,000 per month. Social Security gave me $675 per month, explaining that the low amount was because I hadn't paid a lot in taxes.

At this point, I was 27 and, because I couldn't afford the insurance, I had to get rid of my faithful truck. Looking on the bright side, I was now afforded the opportunity to concentrate on my recovery.

I also had a DUI charge to tend to, from that incident in which I had crashed into a metal barrier. Luckily, I was represented by an able public defender. In court, he took me into a private room where I remember telling him that I didn't think I had had any alcohol to drink that day. He "side-barred" a discussion with the judge, after which the prosecutor announced, "Prosecutor withdraws the case for no evidence."

All the other defendants in the courtroom roared in applause as if they were hungry for a defense victory.

My mother, to help in any way she could, moved me in with her in Florida, where I had plenty of time to reflect on my condition. I felt like I had landed in a whole new body with limits I wasn't used to.

What was wrong with me, I thought as I meditated on my situation. Why can't I do the things that I used to find so easy?

My mental chemistry was so out of balance that I had to remain silent most of the time, because even a regular conversation caused me an unbearable amount of anxiety. My life was totally unnatural. Friends of the family would soon be visiting, and I wondered if I would even be able to talk to them.

To begin handling my condition, I had to live an extremely calm life. Metaphorically speaking, the paralysis of my mind was similar to the paralysis of one's legs. Environmental stimulation could easily leave me stressed out.

Will I ever begin to DJ again? It's impossible.

I spent my days secluded in my bedroom, listening to classical music and attempting to read abstract books about the law. Although I was off a little, I had an insatiable craving to acquire useful information. I knew I would never be able to handle law school, so I decided to try paralegal studies. My local community college had a nice paralegal program online, and I began to get high grades in my courses.

I quickly realized, however, that reading boring case law all day wasn't creative enough to be my life purpose. Furthermore, if I made one single mistake in the law, it could cause a malpractice suit against my employer. Learning the law became so stressful that, although I gained new respect for lawyers who put themselves through it all, I discontinued my paralegal studies.

By this time, my medication was so strong that I was sleeping twelve to sixteen hours every day. My mother, who had her own mental disabilities, thought my sleeping so much was due to laziness. She grew tired of having to assist me as an adult and longed for the days when her childcare would again be over. She and I got into regular arguments, during which she would call the police, who would have to explain to her that there was nothing they could do if nothing illegal had happened.

My breaking point came when my mother got a boyfriend, who infested the apartment with fleas from his farm dog. I could literally see them dancing around the apartment. Before I knew it, my mother left town with the guy and the dog, but left the fleas behind, making the apartment insufferable.

Larissa and her husband, John, loathed my mom's unforgiving attitude toward my condition, so they invited me to stay with them. John talked me into stealing household items from my mom on my move out, explaining that Florida law made that easy to get away with. (I eventually gave my mom back everything I could. We forgave each other, and everything worked out in the long run. She's still a great mom.) John was initially very compassionate about my stay in his home, taking me out to family dinners.

By this time, I had been taking medications for years, and their healing effect slowly increased my wellness. A doctor once told me that would happen.

"The longer you take medication for schizophrenia," he said, "the more you gradually progress in your recovery."

New Opportunities

Soon after I moved out of my mom's apartment, the miracle of this slow recovery began to afford me the privilege of starting to DJ again. I found within myself the passion to give my DJ performances everything I had. I would spend countless hours downloading music and getting back into the nightclub scene a little bit at a time. Knowing this was my life purpose, I was so happy that I found something I loved to spend my time on. I will say here that I didn't drink alcohol or take drugs, and still don't, because that's why my father committed suicide.

I loved visiting my therapist; she had a doctorate in psychology. In therapy, I relearned how to work by taking tasks one at a time, so they didn't become too stressful. Also, I pursued one nightclub at a time, so I didn't have too much on my plate at once. As a result, I gradually got back into working.

Although I had years of previous experience as a DJ in Pennsylvania, I decided to intern to learn the advancements in the field and get my foot in the door in

Florida. One of my best internships came from the local radio station's very own club DJ, whom I will call Sidney, who had a pretty big name for himself locally. After hearing him, I fell in love with his mainstream DJing style. He had absolutely no clue who I was, and yet he offered to help me during his residency at Blue Martini Lounge.

Success at last!

His humility and willingness to take me under his wing took me back. I considered him the second-best DJ I'd ever heard, so being coached by him was a dream come true.

I also built a relationship with a well-known local DJ whom I will call Jason. The club where he spun had a big room that could hold a crowd of 300 or more. Although people faulted him for playing too much of the same music, he gave me lots of useful insights from his fourteen years of live DJ experience. He slowly increased my live DJ time, controlling my every move. Having to DJ everything *his way,* almost record for record, was stressful, but it was worth having such a big venue on my resumé. And eventually, he gave me freedom to play my own sets. Amazingness!

Jason wanted me to take the initiative to break up fights during those crazy nights. One time, it took everything I had to try to hold a huge guy back from practically killing someone, but there was nothing I could do about it. He appeared to be on steroids, and his punches were deadly blows to the other guy's ribs, over and over again in the same spot. It turned out that the guy who had been beaten up was going around with a friend and flirting with everyone's girlfriends.

The best moment of all was watching a provocative obese old man dancing on stage as he rubbed his nipples through his shirt to put on a show. The good thing about a hole-in-the-wall venue is that the atmosphere makes people feel more comfortable to let their hair down and not care if anyone is watching.

When word spread that the area's biggest nightclub was closing, big DJs came out of the woodwork to ask Jason if they could DJ there before it went out of business. Since Jason liked working with me, he had me DJ instead of another guy, who had live on-air experience from radio station HOT 97 in New York.

The grand closing was something amazing to be a part

of. The radio station's MC offered to work for free, and Jason played a nostalgic music video of people waving to the camera, consisting of footage that he had captured since the club's doors opened. At the end of the night, various people spoke about the emotional closing, and all the guests signed their names on the wall before leaving. At least a thousand people stopped by in the course of the night.

Around this time, I started dating a girl I will call Jess. I was taken by the fact that she had a big heart and did everything she could to help me, which immediately won me over. When I moved in with her and her three-year-old daughter, Elizabeth, John got angry because he was used to getting money from me for rent. Afterward, he began claiming that I owed him back payments.

Why didn't he say anything to me previously?

He locked me out of the garage and kept my sentimental tool collection, telling my aunt that he was holding my tools in lieu of the rent money. Before this, John had always responded to my texts, but now he never did. I was upset for a long time because I had been slowly building the tool collection since I was a little kid. In fact, the tools were a part of me.

As I began a spiritual journey with Jess, I realized that letting go of material things is essential to the well-being of someone suffering.

A few months after I moved in with Jess, we got married—I guess a bit too hastily, because right after I married her, she became abusive toward me. At least once or twice a month, she would attack me physically. But it wasn't the physical abuse that bothered me most. It was the verbal abuse. Practically every conversation we had ended with her being verbally confrontational. I learned that no matter how genuine and warm I was, I couldn't salvage a relationship if my partner was violent.

Because of the unhealthy relationship I had with Jess, my sisters, Larissa and Linda, came to believe that Jess was using me for my Social Security and cheating on me with another guy.

After this, I performed my own little investigation of Jess, and found out that she never cheated on me and she was going into debt with me, so she couldn't be using me for my Social Security. This made me realize that my sisters could accuse someone of something unfairly. This situation reminded me of the saying by Steven Covey, author of *The 7 Habits of Highly Effective People*, who said, "Seek first to understand, then to be understood."[4]

Some of my life's greatest blessings came from this completely dysfunctional relationship with Jess. Here's how that started: Since Jess took advice only from her psychic friends, she consulted one of them about me and was told that if I created a savings account, I would start to get more DJ work. In fact, that's just what happened. Receiving such accurate advice from someone who never met me sent chills down my spine. Over a short period of time, psychics proved themselves to me, earned my confidence, and usually turned out to be right.

Another thing that opened the door to my miraculous spiritual path was experiencing Reiki, an ancient Asian healing technique, firsthand. Reiki practitioners take loving, healing energy from a "Source"—whether God, Buddha, Jesus, angels, nature, or whatever—channel it into their own body, and then send it on to another person, animal, tree, or anything else that needs healing. The loving energy heals everything it comes into contact with,

[4]New York: Simon & Schuster, 1989, p. 247.

eventually driving out negative energy.

For the first month of receiving Reiki, I was sad, as I re-experienced all the negative energy in my body that I had accumulated over the years. After my body finished purging the negative energy, Reiki started to make me feel amazing each time. Among other things, today it is an accepted form of cancer treatment in hospitals.

When Jess first took me to her Reiki master, I asked to be calmed down, since my biggest problem at the time was anxiety. When we meditated together before the session, I felt that I was going to pass out, but the master talked me into receiving Reiki, saying that she would stop if anything adverse happened. Then she really got into it, doing breathwork and everything.

As Jess and I were driving away, the healing effect of Reiki was transforming. The only thing I can compare it to is the complete blissful calmness I had experienced as a very young child. Modern medicine has never made me feel this perfectly healthy form of calmness. Fifteen minutes of calming Reiki was so powerful that it had a healing effect that lasted for three days.

I have since learned that psychics have a way of

directly communicating with heavenly sources to give people guidance in the present about the future. At one point, I spent a whole morning desperately asking angels for help because God hadn't seemed to answer a prayer of mine in years. In fact, I was starting to wonder if God even existed. My request of the angels was for them to send Jess's channeler friend a message to make Jess stop abusing me.

When Jess came home, she sat down at the foot of the bed, where I was lying down. As I sat up, I saw a small sparkle of white light twist through the air.

I thought I might have been seeing things, but Jess said, "Did you see that?"

"Yes," I said.

"That's what an angel looks like!" she said.

Her words sent shivers down my spine because I had been desperately asking the angels to help me right before she sat down. Since we both saw the same sparkle of light, I knew it was real.

My inspiration to learn about angels came about because whenever I called on them, I would see a shimmer of light fly through the air, and my situations would magically fix themselves. I was so inspired that Jess and I went to the library to find the perfect book about angels. Ironically, that book, *Archangels and Ascended Masters* by Doreen Virtue, a spiritually enlightened psychologist with a doctorate in psychology, turned out to be on display at the end of the aisle.[5] I didn't even have to look for it. Seemingly, it found me.

Before bed every night, I would read about a few spiritual beings and call upon them for help, just to see what happened. I remember reading somewhere about how angels can show us signs through electronic messages. The first night I read the book, I called upon the goddess Abundantia to ask for good fortune and to confirm that she had received my request. I was hoping she would bring about new financial opportunities for me.

When I tuned into the meditation Pandora station on my cell phone to go to sleep, an electronic advertisement popped up immediately, saying, "Opens New Doors . . . DeVry University." So that is how the Divine speaks

---

[5]Doreen Virtue, *Archangels and Ascended Masters: A Guide to Working and Healing with Divinities and Deities* (Carlsbad, CA: Hay House, 2003).

through signs. That was also the type of confirmation I was learning about, so I knew in my heart that this experience was real. I smiled to myself and went to sleep.

I also recall asking Archangel Raguel for some "life justice," because he is known to help underdogs.

Will this pathway eventually lead me back to God? What is going to happen to my future career?

These were all mysteries that I had in my mind as I took this journey.

By this time in my life, the mental handicap portion of my schizophrenia had greatly improved. Although I still experienced some anxiety, I was now dealing mainly with the side effects of my medications. Most of all, I was still sleeping too much. But my sense of reality was intact, so I don't want the reader to believe that my experiences with angels were just the products of hallucination.

In any case, Jess made me aware that Native American psychics have found that everyone has past family members who help them in the spiritual dimension. They call these beings "spirit guides." In this connection, Jess taught me a secret of the universe. I could meet my guardian angels and spirit guides, she said, if I meditated and asked them to step forth and say their names. She emphasized that I should stay neutral and not force any messages to come through. The act of communicating like this is known as channeling. If any of my readers think channeling isn't real, they can easily find books on the subject at any New Age bookstore.

How amazing!

In any case, I couldn't wait to try it!

So I sat on my bed that night, filled with anticipation, and thought, *Guardian angels, please step forth and say your names.*

I received their messages by seeing words in white letters and hearing words in my mind's ear. (Psychic communication is different for everyone. Some people hear the message, see it, or just somehow know what it is.[6])

An angel's name came through as gibberish, which looked something like this:

Wasistboevignqauclrnosrhenmaolemaifjewmcne

---

[6]See Doreen Virtue, *Angel Therapy: Healing Messages for Every Area of Your Life* (Carlsbad, CA: Hay House, 1997).

I later learned that angels' heavenly names are not meant to be said by human tongues. When I paused in my meditation to let my spirit guides come forth and say their names, I heard the name *Ralph* uttered very loudly, and felt that I was being connected to something extremely powerful, for Ralph was my maternal grandfather. Then I heard the name *Eddie*, said more softly and naturally. Eddie was my father. After hearing those names, I thanked the angels and spirit guides for stopping by and ended my meditation.

I must note here that if you try this for yourself, you should ask God to oversee that you're communicating to the right beings and that He's protecting you. There are other beings in the spiritual dimension that can prank you or prey on your fears.[7] You can call upon God to help you at *any* time.

If you call on angels for help, it is worth noting that they can divide into billions of identical beings. Just like God, they can help billions of people at the same time. You also don't have to know which angel to call upon for

---

[7]Sanaya Roman and Duane Packer, *Opening to Channel: How to Connect with Your Guide* (Tiburon, CA: H. J. Kramer, 1987).

your situation. They all communicate with each other instantly. All you have to do is think *Angels help me*, and the right angels for the job will instantly be by your side.[8]

Furthermore, angels are a constant source of love, support, respect, and help. There's never a reason to be afraid that they will tire of helping you. They don't need rest because they don't have human bodies. Their reward for helping you is to watch you get better. Divine beings go by the principle that helping you with love is soothing, since we are all connected. Thank them, but know they will always be there for you with loving support. That angels even exist is a miracle in itself.[9]

At that point in my spiritual development, I was calling upon angels and general spiritual beings for help. Calling upon angels was a starting point for me, because I was too afraid to call upon God. However, the Bible states that God is the highest being in the universe, and the angels serve Him and Jesus.

I analyzed meeting my spirit guides a million times after that first meditation to think through if it was real or a

---

[8]Virtue, *Angel Therapy*.
[9]Virtue, *Angel Therapy*.

figment of my imagination. If my brain had been making up the responses, I would have seen the words *Dad* or *Grandpop*, because that's what I called them. I believed in my heart that it was they who were speaking to me, because they told me that their names were Ralph and Eddie. Also, I *never* had thoughts come into my head in white letters before. I have only experienced thinking in white letters when I channel, which is completely different from my regular thinking. The white letters made it legitimate for me.

After taking the advice of Jess's psychic to create a savings account that would remove my spiritual block to receiving DJ work, a big lead came though on my online booking account.

Was this also because I requested help from Abundantia and Raguel?

This was a high-energy concert for a Color Run to be attended by thousands of people. This Color Run was a 5K party with a charitable contribution. The participants got up at 8:00 A.M., ran a 5K, and came back to my concert at the stage. During the concert, there were countdowns when the participants released vibrant color powder packets into the air. That was *so* liberating.

At that time, the thought of taking on a crowd of several thousand people was a bit overwhelming, so I almost turned the gig down. However, Jess encouraged me to take it because we were poverty-stricken, and I had to provide for the family.

I had to hire a full-time MC to work with me, so I happily brought Sidney to the show, which was a dream come true. The performance went ten times better than I had imagined, so we began traveling all over Florida, performing concerts for thousands of people. It was an amazing feeling to be so successful, which inspired me to look forward to much larger events.

Fortunately for me, Jess refused to acknowledge that I was disabled. Insisting that I was perfectly normal, she pushed me to ascend to high levels of responsibility and functionality, putting me on a path that would take me far beyond anything I had ever dreamed possible.

Sandalphen at a Bowling Alley

Jason asked me to fill in for him during his DJ residency in an upscale bowling alley. During that time, I was lacking inspiration. On my way there, I was intently asking Archangel Sandalphen to inspire me. As soon as I walked in, I heard "Angel of Mine" by Toni Braxton playing on the Internet radio station. At first, I thought, *Huh, what a grand coincidence. "Angel of Mine" never plays on the radio anymore, anywhere.*

At that point, I knew that Sandalphen was with me. Then he spoke to my situation by playing the next song, "Take Back the Night" by Justin Timberlake. The message for me to take back the night through my DJ'ing was very empowering. No one was aware that this series of miracles had just happened to me. However, I was so inspired that I DJ'd as if there were no tomorrow! One teenage boy who worked at the bowling alley actually came up to me to say that I was one of the best DJs he had ever heard there.

I went home and fell asleep for the night, and the next morning I explained my experience from the bowling alley to Jess in our family room, who pointed at the sliding glass door.

"Archangel Raphael's shows me his emerald energy next to that door all the time. He likes to hang out here."

That's interesting, why can't I ever see him?

Abuse

On the other hand, although Jess helped me to recover, her physical and mental abuse began to take a heavy toll on me. It seemed that she was always fighting me over the slightest details, which sometimes led her into raging physical abuse. Her psychic friends said that since Jess's energy and mine were combined through marriage, she must be taking on my lower past-life karma. That led me to believe that my whole life was destined for suffering.

The very first time Jess attacked me physically, we had gotten into an argument over something, so I ran into the bathroom and locked her out. But she kicked the door open and ran toward me as if she were going to kill me. I stepped out of the way, which caused her to crash into a huge pile of laundry. At that point, she kept yelling at me, but stopped her physical attack. I hoped—wrongly, as it turned out—that I would never see that kind of violence from her again.

Unfortunately, that was only the first of several such

incidents. On many occasions, she came clawing for my throat over trivial arguments, sometimes leaving marks on my neck. I'm sure she often had my skin under her nails afterward. Whenever she got that way, I had to take her seriously because, although she was smaller than me, her rage could make her as strong as a man.

After so many months of this torture, I started to research ways to commit suicide, and thought of throwing myself under the train that went by, a block away, every night. I also prayed intently for God to end my life in my sleep. Those were moments of deep emotional suffering.

(Play Led Zeppelin's "When the Levee Breaks.")

One night, when I was researching statistics on suicide methods, three-year-old Elizabeth came up to me and said something so sweet that it was impossible to bring myself to go through with my plans. She had such a healing force in just a few short words. That is the miraculous healing power that children can have on us.

However, one night I reached my breaking point. Falling to my knees, I begged God for mercy from Jess's combative abuse. At moments like that, I also ask St. John to make me cry to help me heal. The more passionately you pray for something, they say, the more passionately the Divine answers. After I prayed that night, the most incredible thing happened.

As I dreamt in my sleep, everything cleared into a deep black space, as if it were the universe before everything was created. It looked like a panoramic view of existence. God appeared as a golden shade of white light that took up nearly the entire panorama. When I wondered what His presence felt like, He paused the dream to send me a sense of calmness and a touch of happiness. Then a flash of white light suddenly burst out of Him, passing between planets and heading toward Earth. The light literally struck me on the head, knocking me off the couch to the floor. However, I managed to land on my feet and laughed at the idea that God had just slapped me awake. Then another series of miracles occurred.

First, when I hit the floor, I was instantly completely awake, as if I had been up for hours. That was a miracle, because due to the side effects of my medications, it usually took me four hours to become that awake.

Second, I knew God was present because when I sat down at my desk, the phone immediately rang with a call from a new DJ client. That timing was more perfect than a movie director could have created. It has been said that God is in your presence when things happen with perfect timing. This whole series of events was a mind-boggling mystery to me. *Why did God come into my dreams, and why did He wake me up with a bolt of light to my head?* For the life of me, I couldn't figure that out. God certainly works in mysterious ways.

*

One day, Jess threatened that if I ever spoke to my sisters again I would have to "get the fuck out."

That night, she tested my limits for tolerating abuse. As she got angrier and angrier over almost nothing, she suddenly grabbed the footlong, razor-sharp kitchen knife and emphasized each point by pushing the knife toward my face.

Now, let me pause my story for a moment. I had to stop and think about this as it was happening. When Jess got mad like that, she became as strong as a man. Therefore, I had to take her threatening gestures very seriously.

Could she snap and potentially kill me with that knife?

When I realized that the answer was yes, I knew my life was in danger, and I only had two choices. Either I reached for the knife and fought to disarm her, or I played it cool and hoped she left me alone. I decided to play it cool. Fortunately, after yelling at me some more, she went into the kitchen to cut up some vegetables.

After a moment, I followed her into the kitchen.

"I didn't do anything to deserve that," I said.

That earned me a bowl of spaghetti and meatballs in my face. Then she planted her feet like a boxer, clenched her fist, and threw the best right hook of her life.

Now, the reader should know that I had been on my high-school wrestling team, with my stepdad, Josh, as my personal coach. Josh was not just any wrestler. He entered the wrestling hall of fame for winning two state championships in scholastic wrestling and three world championships in freestyle wrestling. In fact, he would have made it into the Olympics if he hadn't gotten into trouble with the law. During my high-school years, he had me wrestling state champions. I wasn't the greatest wrestler in the world, but I did train with the best.

So, as Jess swung at me, I simply stepped back, and she completely missed me. The swing was so powerful that it probably would have knocked me out if it had connected, and taken three of my teeth with it.

Is she capable, I wondered, *of understanding what's going wrong with our marriage?*

I decided to test her awareness of how crazy things had become by giving her a small smack to her cheek. I wouldn't have hurt a fly, but I needed to make her realize what she was doing, and stop.

Will she then snap out of it?

No.

I had left the food she shoved in my face there to show her what she had just done, but it didn't seem to have any effect on her. It was clear that there was nothing in the whole world that would ever make her realize how out of control things had become. There was absolutely nothing in my power to fix her abusive state of mind. After six short months, I realized that my marriage was completely irreparable.

I knew I was in a vulnerable position, because she knew how to manipulate the law so that she could attack me physically and then have me thrown in jail by lying to the cops that *I* had attacked *her*. Florida's domestic violence laws seem to be slanted against men.

When I realized that, I headed straight for the front door, leaving all of my possessions behind, including my expensive DJ equipment, not caring if she destroyed it all. The only thing that mattered to me at that moment was to leave.

But there was nowhere for me to go—no emergency homeless shelters in the area, and no public housing to take me in. My sister Linda was the only one I could call, but that meant giving up Jess. Nevertheless, I called her, and she picked me up and graciously gave me a place to stay. I felt so calm leaving in my sister's car.

"I *knew*," she said, "that Jess has been abusing you all this time. In fact, I even went to the police about it. They told me that she had driven her mild-mannered ex-husband to fire a gun in the house."

That gave me an eerie feeling that I had been sleeping next to an abusive woman this whole time and never knew it until I married her.

Linda said, "The police told me to wait till you got sick

of the abuse and needed a place to stay. 'You can bet,' they said, 'he'll be calling you one of these days.'"

After I left the house, I realized I had an edge to me that night, and that turned out to be the answer to my prayers to fix my situation and the reason for God's mystery dream the night before. In other words, I realized that God had come into my dream to say, "Hey, I'm answering your prayer." He woke me up just early enough to give me the edge that it took to leave Jess that night. It was a small miracle and the reason for the flash of light that woke me up so quickly.

Just before I moved into Linda's apartment, she said to me, "You can stay rent free, save your money, and then get a place of your own. You can use my car for important appointments, too."

I feel so blessed!!

Savannah

(Play two songs back to back: "Twist and Shout" by the Beatles and "She's Got a Way" by Billy Joel.)

Around this time, I was completely finished with Jess, feeling the need for a genuine partner, and that's when I asked my guardian angel to bring me Savannah. My angel advised me on how to court Savannah, which gave me confidence that my soon-to-be dream girl would be mine in the long run. So, I only cared about giving her my love, not receiving anything in return. In the end, I completely swept her off her feet by healing her with Reiki. After that, it became common for us to heal each other.

On one occasion, when I was walking to the corner store for a snack, I asked my angel to speak to me through music as I listened to a Pandora station on my cell phone. My angel played "Beautiful People" by Benni Benassi and Chris Brown, which sent a very clear message to me. My angel was telling me to just be my beautiful self, and Savannah would like me as I was. Thus, there was no need to try to impress her.

Savannah was the only girl I ever *loved* who could reject me without hurting my feelings. One time, I channeled her grandmother, who was her spirit guide, asking her for a special word that would relate to Savannah's life. The word turned out to be *dream.* The next day, when I was in an arts and crafts store, I ironically came across a wooden sculpture that spelled out the word *dream.*

However, when I gave it to Savannah, she said, "Is this road kill, or *what*?"

I liked her so much that I thought that was cute.

Because of the medications I was on for schizophrenia, my sleep patterns were disrupted, so I often kept Savannah up for hours on the phone, late at night. We connected on every level, and quickly realized that we were perfect for each other. As soon as we realized we had something going for each other, we stayed very loyal and completely committed to each other, leaving our previous relationships in the past.

Savannah was everything I ever wanted in a woman. In fact, we had so much in common that I regarded her as me in female form. We eventually went on to have a John Lennon and Yoko Ono type of love.

Enfolded in Angel Wings

One night at Linda's before going to bed, I was trying to cope with the abuse I faced from Jess, and I pondered what it would be like to be enfolded in angel wings. So as I lay in my bed before going to sleep, I started to meditate. After about a minute or so I requested that my guardian angel wrap its wings around me.

I began to feel a calm, gentle energy surrounding me. After a few moments, the surrounding energy became a gentle warm blanket and I went to sleep very peacefully.

Our First Meditation Together

Savannah and I grew trust early on, and she decided that she wanted to try her first meditation with me.

I suggested that we have our guardian angels give us this experience. We lay down as we spoke over the phone, and I began guiding us through the meditation.

After walking us through each step, I said, "Now it is time for our angels to send us any messages they would like us to know."

A few minutes passed, and after concluding the meditation, I asked Savannah,

"Did you receive any visualizations from your guardian angel?"

"Yes!!" she replied.

"What happened?? Tell me!"

"I was walking through an enchanted forest that was so magical! The trees had faces and could speak. When I got to the end of the trail, there was a beautiful, large wedding chapel."

"Did it look like this?" I said.

I messaged her pictures of the Vatican.

"Yes, it looked just like that!" she said.

"I always wanted to get married there," I said.

"You have to be a Catholic and conform to their religion for that to happen," she said.

"Since I am spiritual, not of any sect, I guess they wouldn't let me," I said.

We laughed.

"When I did my first meditation with my angel, he took me on a flying adventure with him!" I said.

Then we decided to retire until the next day.

Dreaming

A few nights later, just before I went to sleep, I asked the Divine and God to make sure I received my new DJ headphones in the mail before my next Color Run that weekend. I fell fast asleep, and that morning, while I was dreaming, I began to see white letters that showed the word, "Delivery." The letters suddenly faded away and the cell phone next to my physical body rang at once. I woke up with a feeling someone was trying to get in touch with me.

"Hello?"

"Hey, I'm the FedEx driver with a delivery for you, I just don't know which apartment is yours."

I ran out in perfect timing to catch the delivery driver driving by. After receiving the delivery, I realized the Divine actually does know where everyone is, and what they are doing, all at once. Then I realized that my prayer to receive my headphones on time had been directly answered.

The Divine has a superior technology to pull something

like this off so perfectly!

Oh, Boy

Unfortunately, Linda's roof started leaking, and she grew worried that her landlord would find me there and charge her more money for rent. Also, since the apartment only had two bedrooms, I had to sleep in her daughter Kristin's bed, while Kristin slept with Linda. Kristin, who was five, kicked in her sleep, so the stress of my stay became quickly amplified for my sister.

I acknowledged these concerns to Linda, and when things started to get really intolerable after three months, I agreed to move out as soon as I could. In the meantime, whenever she asked me to clean a room, I would clean the whole apartment, to show my loving appreciation. I also wrote Linda a heartfelt handwritten note to tell her what an amazing sister she was for giving me a place to stay.

But all that was to no avail, since Linda had started to become verbally abusive. For example, I used the Internet to download music for my DJ career, so she screamed at me one day, "I've turned off the Internet, I'm gonna have the electricity disconnected, and I'm moving outta here!"

I left her apartment in tears, until she called to tell me that she had put all my belongings outside. Apparently, she didn't care if everything got destroyed in the rain—which in Florida can come at any time.

When Linda put all my stuff outside, everyone started to avoid me, so I knew she had told people lower things about me. That made it almost impossible for me to get a place to stay. I know that she told Savannah that I had tried to blow my head off with dynamite, which wasn't true. It was just an abusive attempt to make my twin flame fear dating a schizophrenic.

Savannah wanted to give me a place to stay, but she couldn't because she was living with her mother at the time. Since I didn't want to be homeless, I realized that I had no other option, at least for the moment, than to move back in with Jess.

Back with Jess

In the few months since I had last seen Jess, she had gotten help for her abusiveness and seemed now like a totally different person.

"The doctors said I had a problem with my thyroid," she said.

When I contacted her, she promised that I could sleep on her couch for six months until I could get on my feet and move out.

During this second time that I lived with Jess, I had another amazing spiritual experience that I want to share with the reader. I learned from *angel-guide.com* that there are different choirs in the hierarchy of angels.[10] One of those choirs is called the Seraphim. According to Isaiah 6, they have six wings each and fly above God. How interesting!

Another choir is called the Cherubs, who are said to be pure love and are commonly portrayed as baby angels. I

---

[10]*www.angel-guide.com/hierarchy-angels.html/.*

was relentlessly curious to know what it feels like to be a Cherub in Heaven, so one night, as I went to sleep on the couch, I asked the Cherubs to make me feel what they experience in Heaven. When I closed my eyes, I started feeling my soul rise up. I assumed the Cherubs were taking my soul so high that it extended beyond Earth into Heaven. As I observed with my "inner eyes,"[11] my soul looked like the side of a skyscraper. Then it seemed to form tubes in the center, through which the Cherubs sent a feeling down to me that felt like calming love with a little bit of seriousness. That feeling quickly filled my entire being. It was amazing! At that stage of my growth, I was certain that there was far more to spirituality than many people think.

The moment after this experience ended, I received a message from the Cherubs telling me that life has no limits—absolutely anything is possible. It was such an inspiring message that it changed my life. I felt that, from their view up in Heaven, the Cherubs obviously knew something that I didn't, so I believed what they had to tell me.

[11]Virtue, *Angel Therapy*, p. 163.

During this time, I was affirming to manifest my future. For those of you who don't know, people who manifest are asking the universe to bring something to them. Many people believe that God is the universe, so asking the universe for something is the same as asking God for it. I was taught that affirming is like prayer with extra power behind it.

When you affirm something, you are simply thinking about it, and God will bring it into your future. If you meditate on what you are affirming, it is more powerful than just thinking about it. When you meditate, you can picture yourself in every step you want to take that gets what you want. Then you conclude by affirming that you already have it. The process can be done by visualizing each step. You want to feel the positive emotions you would feel when you receive what you are meditating for. Doing so will make the affirmation stronger and more positive.

For example, if you want to manifest a car, you would meditate by picturing yourself working at a perfect job, and experience what it feels like to be happily successful. Then imagine your savings growing and how happy you would be about receiving them. Next, see yourself selecting your vehicle and feeling good about driving it home.

When the Cherubs told me that life is limitless, I began to affirm limitless things. Why ask for a little when you can ask for everything? If the concept of affirming resonates with you, I encourage you to set your affirmations for the stars. Build a relationship with God and the angels, since they are the universe. If you know that what you are asking for is in alignment with your real-life purpose, they will be happy to help you in the most loving ways possible.

As human beings, we commonly see each other as sinful, but angels see us and treat us all as perfect children of God. They believe that all people are already doing the best they can, and heavenly beings admire us for that. Heavenly beings know that a lifetime on Earth is not always easy. They also look favorably upon us for the bravery we have to accept this challenge in our lifetime.

The next time I spoke to Jess, we began talking about spiritual things, and she said that her spirit guides had informed her that part of my life purpose is to help people with their spiritual lives.

Huh? I thought. *How is that going to come about?*

Although Jess didn't know about Savannah during my stay this time, once she realized that I wasn't coming back to continue being her husband, she immediately wanted me out again. In other words, she was putting me back on the path to being homeless.

I asked every friend and family member if I could stay with them, but no one would even let me sleep on the floor for a day or two, until I could be accepted into a homeless shelter. Linda had apparently made up so many low things about me that everyone turned their back on me. DJ Jason had an extra bedroom, but he still acted as if my sleeping there for a few days would be a big problem for him.

In any case, Jess kicked me out, and I was back on the street. I had to survive in parks, hoping that I wouldn't get noticed by the police, because being homeless in parts of South Florida is actually illegal. I had to roll up a bath towel to use as a pillow to sleep on a narrow metal park bench, where I could smell the harsh odor of a nearby animal carcass. If a cop saw me and decided to take me to jail, I could have lost my entire DJ career, because the prison intake officers might steal my expensive laptop and hard drives.

The good part about being homeless in that area was being immersed in nature. I could hear the nearby ocean waves from my bench, which was very soothing and healing. I found that sleeping in nature is more healing than I previously realized.

Somehow, Savannah stood by me and supported me in every way she could during this period that I was homeless. Her loving support was unwavering.

On my third night in the park, a cop showed up around 11:00 P.M. to kick me out. The only other park I knew I could sleep in was miles away in a completely different town. My medication required me to sleep twelve hours every night, but because of the hot and humid Florida weather, I was quickly worn down. Nevertheless, I got on my bike in the middle of the night, with all my heavy belongings, and headed for that distant park.

With my energy depleted, I didn't get much sleep at the other park. Furthermore, I had to wake up at 5:00 A.M. and leave before the local park-goers found me there.

When I got up at dawn and rode my bike back into

town, I burned up every last drop of my strength. As I peddled down a road that ran along the beach. I had to stop three times to sleep on the hot sand in the scorching sun, because that was the only place I could find to rest. I got eaten by fire ants, but was too tired to fight them off. I was also fighting hunger. Eventually, I made it to a Dunkin' Donuts, where I refueled with a bagel and half a bottle of Smartwater, all that I could afford. I was totally desperate, but held back my tears.

When a woman in the donut shop noticed how sad I looked, she told me about three local churches that might help me. I was completely elated to hear that there was a church nearby that provided housing for homeless people. That news brought me so much joy that I found some motivation within myself to continue on just a little further.

After getting lost for a while, I finally found the church and prayed that it could help me, because I had nowhere else to go. As it happened, a social function at the church was just ending, and when I humbly approached people who were walking out, they encouraged me to talk to the priest.

However, the people in charge refused to let me talk to the priest, insisting that I leave immediately. One elderly man stretched out his thick arthritic fingers, grabbed my shoulder, and walked me out of the church. I couldn't understand why I was being treated this way, since I was very calm and appreciative. I was sensing darkness in the situation.

Knowing I had no energy left to ride my bike anywhere else, I called a pastor who had given me counseling a few years earlier, telling him that I was literally shaking and ready to collapse on the ground. When he advised me to ride across town to another church, I told him that was impossible for me, since I could hardly stand up anymore. Unfortunately, he had other plans, so he could not give me a ride.

By the grace of God, I managed to ride my bike back to the Dunkin' Donuts just in time to collapse on their outdoor bench. As I cried my eyes out, I dialed 911 and lay there helplessly until an ambulance came to get me.

As the paramedic approached me, his facial expression and body language seemed repelled by my tears. He acted as if helping me was doing some kind of favor to the community.

"Is this your shit?" he said, pointing to my bags, as he avoided helping me up. But another emergency medical technician helped me into the back of the ambulance, where I rode to a small local hospital.

When I got there, I was taken care of by a male nurse practitioner, who treated me with respect. In the freezing cold hospital, he took a warm blanket from a dryer and floated it over me.

As I lay on the bed, the nasty EMT walked into the room for a moment to get something he had forgotten. When he noticed my half-empty bottle of Smartwater, he looked at me as if to say, "If you can drink something with electrolytes in it, what are you doing in a hospital?" Then, on his way out, he shook his head as if my problems were what was wrong with *his* life.

A little later, the nurse practitioner came in to discharge me.

"Mister Faggioli," he said, "you had heatstroke. Take these potassium pills, and you can go."

When I called Jess to tell her what had happened, she regretted that her throwing me into the street had caused this, so she agreed to let me sleep on her couch again until I could get myself into a homeless shelter—hopefully as quickly as possible. Fortunately, she still had no idea about Savannah.

Three days later, when I had regained some of my strength, I called Christ Fellowship, the biggest church in the area, to ask if they took in homeless people. The pastor I spoke to, who prayed passionately with me on the phone, told me that the only nearby shelter that had any room was a few towns away and only took in three or four new people every day. Therefore, I had to wake up early every morning, still tired from my medication, and call for three days before there was an opening. It was Easter time, so one might think that shelters would be more charitable than usual in rescuing people, but in fact there were more homeless folks competing for the spaces.

During the night before my move, when I was packing for the homeless shelter, Jess became abusive again, telling me that I couldn't use her washing machine because she didn't want to pay for the water. To put that problem into perspective for her, I offered her a dollar for the four cents of water I would use. But she turned me down.

“You can wash your clothes where you’re going,” she said.

Then she switched off the lamp that was lighting the living room, and said to me in the moonlight that was coming in the window, “I’m not paying for your electricity, either!”

“Don’t you think that’s abusive?” I said. “How am I gonna pack if I can’t see what I’m doing?”

Since she was making a monumental spiritual effort to change for the better, she said, “Fine. You can use that one light. And then go to sleep!”

The Beginning of No Return

Getting into the shelter was a small miracle in itself. However, the place, which was in a rundown part of town in the projects, had an industrial feel to it and turned out to be very unhealthy. To begin with, the food, which came from the local jail, was inedible. I confined myself to peanut butter and jelly sandwiches. One evening, the chicken that was being served for dinner looked so slimy that it literally turned my stomach. I totally avoided it, but all the residents who ate it got diarrhea.

There were twelve women residents on the ground floor, housed three to a room, and twenty men on the second floor, housed the same way. The two sexes were kept totally separate, except for classes—which mostly had to do with anger management, budgeting, and resumé writing. The anger classes were redundant because I had just spent almost seven years exhausting a therapist on that topic.

Like most other shelters in South Florida, this one was

primarily created for homeless drug addicts. The staff members were aware that I hadn't consumed alcohol in seven years, but they nevertheless forced me attend AA meetings every week. Otherwise, I would have to leave. With only three months to get a job and move out, I was driven crazy by the way they pressured me to attend AA and other meetings, which kept me from searching for a job.

During my first week at the shelter, I wasn't allowed to leave the premises at all because the staff assumed that I would try to get high on the outside. I also wasn't permitted to have any visitors. Fortunately, starting in the second week, Savannah was allowed to pick me up, but I had to meet her across the street.

When I asked why, the caseworker replied, "We don't want any homeless murderers on the property."

One evening, I was lying on my single-sized mattress looking at the wall and reflecting on life. As my vision relaxed, it was as if I could somehow see the energy moving through the floor and up the wall. *Is it true that we can actually see energy this way?* That question in my mind wanted to be answered, but I didn't know anyone who could.

The following night, I was in the shelter's AA meeting daydreaming when my vision became unfocused again while looking the speaker. As my vision loosened, it was as if I could see a yellow outline around his body. *Was this his aura,* I thought? In perfect timing, there was a flash of blue light in between him and the window located behind him, as I intuitively could sense that Archangel Michael was responding with a confirming "Yes" to my question.

Knowing this was a judgment-free zone, I went to the speaker after the meeting and said, "When you were speaking, you had an angel near you."

As if I had given him goose bumps, he said, "You know, you're not the first person to approach me and tell me that."

Perhaps more and more people are evolving to see angels these days, I thought.

✶

A few days later, when I was back at the daily grind in the shelter. I thought I might drum up a little DJ work while I was preparing my resumé and listing employment prospects, but my caseworker said, “You can do DJ gigs as long as the director approves an hourly time schedule so she can see that you’re out working and not doing drugs.”

I thought, *I’m a vegan who hardly even drinks caffeine, let alone milk or cheese. But, never mind, I’ll get it done!*

Two days later, I got hired by a nightclub to DJ every Thursday night, which the owner announced on Facebook.

Thank God I would be getting paid to do what I love!

However, when I showed my schedule to my caseworker, she said, “The director didn’t approve of you leaving the shelter.”

“You already told me I could do it,” I said, looking at her with confusion.

“Sorry, you can’t do it.”

I was so upset that I turned around and left the office before I said something I would regret. As I walked into my room, my roommate was just adjusting his tie.

“Where are *you* going?” I asked.

“I’m leaving the shelter for a week of job training.”

“They won’t even let me leave for a DJ gig,” I said. Why are you allowed to go for an entire week?”

"When the shelter did your intake," he said, "did you tell them that you got drunk?"

"Yeah! But that was over seven years ago!"

"That's the reason they treat you like an alcoholic," he said patiently. "They're used to getting lied to when they interview people with addictions."

Now I had the unpleasant task of telling the nightclub owner that I wouldn't be able to DJ for her. Not wanting her to have to scramble for a substitute at the last minute, I called her immediately and told her that something personal had come up. Fortunately, she was very understanding and found someone to fill in for me.

Around this time, I met a fellow resident named Kyle. Most of the other residents went around in tattered clothes, but Kyle was different. He always seemed to be shopping for expensive clothing, but never seemed to be looking for a job.

"Why are you here?" I asked. "You look like you just stepped out of an executive suite."

"I got caught up in some bad Internet business," he said. "I stole someone's identity and my girlfriend kicked me out."

Then, jokingly, he added, "Look at us! We're both homeless because of women! They have no feelings!"

Thinking of Jess, I had to smile.

When I asked Kyle why I couldn't leave the shelter during the first week, he explained that when the state gives money to a homeless shelter, the facility finds a million ways to try to control people, thinking they're all addicts.

"But the rules don't work," he said. "In the long run, the director discovers that she has no control over the residents' addictions. They save up their money, and when they come out, they blow it all away on some alcohol and heroin that they buy down the street. To try to prevent that, these facilities become so burdened with rules that it's like being in a mental hospital."

As in a mental hospital, we were not allowed to have toenail clippers in our possession because we might harm someone or ourselves with them. That was one of the silliest rules, because we could just as easily grab a pen at the front desk and stab someone in the neck—*if* we wanted to. The point is that every move of the residents could not be controlled if the staff wanted to provide a healthy place for them. The countless rules just made everyone miserable—especially those of us who did *not* have an addiction. After a while in that toxic environment, I started to wish I were sleeping in the park again.

One night, I went into the shelter's little garden area to think about what was going on in my life. As I reflected, I began to see that a shelter should help homeless people compassionately. To be homeless is to live through a severe crisis, so why not work to promote healing? Any readers working with homeless shelters, take note. There should actually be counselors, spiritual healers, and a better feedback program to improve the premises. Perhaps there could even be a separate shelter or section for sober homeless people to allow them more freedom.

As intolerable as things were for me in that shelter, I nevertheless decided to make my own small spiritual contribution to it by giving angel-card readings to anyone who was open to receiving them. The card readings only dealt with divine angels. As it turned out, the readings spoke directly to the residents' current situations and became an inspiring source of hope for them.

Whenever someone requested an angel-card reading, I

had my own intuitive way of selecting the cards. First, I would take the deck to the desk next to my bed, which served as my meditation space, sit down, fan the cards out in my hand, and close my eyes. Then, as I ran my index finger along the top edge of the cards, a white angel-light would flash under my eyelids, telling me that the angels wanted me to choose the card that my finger happened to be touching.

During a card reading for one of the residents, the love card came up, which confused him because he was thinking of ending his relationship with his girlfriend. Ironically, a few days later, I noticed him holding hands with a new female resident. I smiled as I recognized that the card's prediction had come true. It was a healing moment.

My birthday, which fell on a Wednesday that year, happened to come during my stay at the shelter. Savannah felt so sad about my being there at such a time that she decided to create a better memory for me.

"When I pick you up on Saturday," she said, "wear a bathing suit under your clothes."

Maybe she was taking me to the beach!

When we got into her truck to drive away from the shelter, she said, "Close your eyes, and don't open them till I tell you."

After twenty minutes, I was dying to know where we were going.

Where could she possibly be taking me?

But whenever I asked her if I could open my eyes yet, she always said, "No! Keep them closed!"

Finally, after half an hour, she parked the car and turned off the engine.

"Okay," she said, "you can open your eyes now!"

When I did, I saw water slides all over, and realized that we were in a water park that I had only passed before, but never been in.

After Savannah bought the tickets and we had changed into our bathing suits, she headed straight for the biggest slide in sight, and we had to climb three or four stories of stairs to get to the top.

When we got there, I said, "Do you wanna go first?"

"No," she said, knowing this was my first time ever on a water slide, "this is your birthday. *You* go first!"

I jumped into the slide full speed. After a moment, I

thought the ride was going to end with me under water, so I held my breath the whole way down. But that turned out to be totally unnecessary.

After that, we went on every slide in the park and had an amazing time. It was such a refreshing escape from the daily madness I was chained to.

We even shared a tube that floated down a calm stretch of water. Being there was so serene and romantic, as if we were the only two people at the park.

When I got back to the shelter that evening, I decided to try to put up with the shelter's toxic rules so I could qualify for its rehousing program. If residents complied with all the shelter's rules for three months, it would reward them by helping them to find an apartment, give them a bed and some furniture, contribute to moving expenses, and pay the first and last month's rent.

That's my reward at the end of the tunnel!

If I found a day job and saved up at least $2,500, the shelter would help me to find an apartment in less than three months, so I looked frantically on the Internet for anything I could do that didn't require experience. The fatiguing side effects of my medications made me sleep for twelve to sixteen hours a day, so that made it hard to find and keep a job.

After sending out a million resumés, I finally landed one interview to sell medical supplies to sick people who were suffering from diabetes, emphysema, sleep apnea, and any condition that required the use of an oxygen tank, a breathing pump, or a catheter.

The woman who interviewed me was very friendly. After asking me several questions, she said, "I like your enthusiasm, which is perfect for a sales job. I'm going to offer you the position for twelve dollars an hour. What do you think?"

"Sure," I said, "I'll accept that."

When I left her office, I was so proud of myself that I could barely wait to call Savannah.

Although the job of selling by phone required me to take a bus and a train for two hours every day each way to and from the office, I was totally dedicated to my work. Since I had to be in bed by 8:00 P.M. and get up at 5:00 A.M., I usually fell asleep on the way to work, but somehow, by the grace of God, always woke up for my stop just in time.

One night after work, wanting to heal myself from my intense lifestyle, I had the amazing idea to meditate and ask every angel in the universe to send me Reiki energy. That turned out to be one of the most incredible experiences of my entire life! There's probably billions, if not trillions, of angels sending out Reiki energy, so requesting it should be on everyone's bucket list. I felt absolutely incredible after that meditation!

I was jumping through all the irritating hoops at the shelter when I suddenly found myself in trouble—and all because of a napkin!

One day, the lunch lady didn't have any paper plates for us at the food window in the cafeteria, so I went behind the serving area to get some napkins to use as plates.

When she saw me, the lunch lady ran up, ripped the napkins out of my hands, and shouted, "Go back out front, and I'll hand you some."

I did what she asked without a problem.

When the lunch lady reported the incident to her superiors, she couldn't bring herself to admit that she had disrespected me, probably fearing that she would get fired because of it. Instead, she lied by telling Susan, the director, that I grabbed her to get the napkins back. The shelter had very strict rules that didn't tolerate any degree of physical violence. So, I got a call later that day, while I was at work, from my caseworker, Lauren.

"Eddie, your stuff is being packed, and you have to vacate the shelter," she said.

"What?" I said. "What are you talking about," I had no clue what was going on.

"The director," Lauren said, "heard about what you did to the lunch lady, and you need to vacate the shelter immediately."

I'm getting kicked out?

"Huh?" I said. "I didn't do anything to the lunch lady."

"You have to talk to the director about the incident, because I can't do anything about it."

When I arrived at the shelter after work, I was totally confused. At the front entrance, the security staff of the shelter were tying trash bags filled with my clothes and belongings.

"Can I speak with the director?" I said.

"You have to talk to Ernie in the office," one of the guards said.

When I talked to Ernie, he called the director and then hung up the phone.

"She's busy at the moment," he said.

How could she possibly be avoiding a crisis of this magnitude?

At that moment, the outside security guard, who was packing my bags in front of the shelter, came into the front office.

"Here's your belongings," he said. "You have to call someone for a ride and leave the premises."

I had nowhere to go. *Forget this!* I thought.

I walked out on the front grass and called the shelter's main number, asking to speak with the director. The security guard in the office answered without knowing it was me calling from just outside the door. He transferred my call to the director, and suddenly she was available.

"Hello?" she answered.

"This is Eddie, and I don't understand why I'm being kicked out," I said, holding back my state of panic.

"You grabbed the lunch lady," she said coldly.

"No, I didn't!"

"Yes, you did!"

"She's lying!"

"No, she's not. I know her, and I know she would *never* lie to me."

"Review the cameras. Interview witnesses! Can't you do that?"

"I don't think there are any cameras facing the staff in the lunchroom."

"Can you walk back and see?"

"No, because of the rules, I have to go by what the lunch lady reported, and there's nothing we can do to keep you here. If you want to protest this, you can move out and then plead your case. But for now you can't be here."

Hearing me begging the director for a place to stay, the security guard came outside and told me that I had to leave. I guess he didn't want the shelter to look poorly if a prospective resident came by, and saw me crying out for a place to stay. Realizing that the shelter had found me guilty without giving me a reasonable opportunity to prove I was innocent, I had to think quickly, so I politely said to the guard that I just needed to call a ride.

"Make sure your ride pulls right into the front parking space here, where we can see them," he said coldly.

I called Savannah, who was just getting off work, and she arrived quickly. The first thing she did after picking me up was drive across the street to a parking lot, so I could call everyone I could think of for help. But no one would help me.

"Eddie," Savannah said, "I don't have much time, and we already know there's no one willing to help you. The only thing you can do is stay at a motel."

Where to Next?

I wanted to move into an apartment if I could, but I only had $900 saved from my sales job, and didn't know if there were any apartments I could move into for such a small amount. The ones I interviewed for wanted the first month's rent plus a security deposit in order to move in. Since no one would help me, my only option was to take a cheap nearby motel room. I had to accept that Savannah was right.

However, as soon as we pulled up to the motel, a million rough construction workers jumped out of the back of a truck and went into the place. It was clear that they lived there, so Savannah and I began to wonder what I was getting myself into, with neighbors like these.

Nevertheless, I moved in. As it turned out, the bus and train route to work took the same amount of time to my job, so that was good. Also, a maid came to clean the room every day, which I didn't have at the shelter. I focused on these small miracles to stay positive, which helped me to elevate my mood to a higher state when I needed it the most.

Perhaps God didn't want me at the shelter. Thank you, God.

I had to get out of that motel because it was eating up all my money. All I needed was $70 more to move into the only available apartment in my price range. But I couldn't find a single family member to lend me that money. Even my Aunt Zelda, who wanted to help, couldn't because she didn't have that kind of money.

And her ex-husband, my Uncle Robert, said, "I gave you two thousand bucks for your DJ speakers, and I'm not giving you any more. I'm getting old, I'm tired, and you're going to have to be homeless."

He seemed to want to be teaching me about responsibility, but this situation was not due to my own lower behaviors or intensions. This was a legitimate emergency.

Does he understand how exhaustingly humid it is during Florida summer nights? Perhaps he didn't hear about my heatstroke. Having to work after tossing and turning all night in the heat and then taking public transportation would not be a working solution.

Luckily, I suddenly realized that my next paycheck was going to be directly deposited into my bank account the next day, so I could stay at the motel for one more night, and then move into the apartment the next day!

Thank God!!

Before I moved in, I checked out the two-story apartment complex during the day, and it seemed decent enough. In any case, it was the *only* place I could live in and still continue commuting to work on public transit without skipping a beat.

The landlady said that there were only two apartments to choose from, but they were both nice, actually. One was on the ground floor, and the other was on the second floor. She recommended the first option, but I didn't want to hear people walking above me while I was trying to sleep at night, so I asked for the second-floor apartment. When I asked to see it, she said it wasn't cleaned yet, but it would be by the time I moved in. Everything seemed okay, so I signed the lease and closed the deal, realizing that this was my only option.

It wasn't until I moved in that I realized that the neighborhood was not as good as it seemed at first. I had looked the place over when everyone was at work. In the evening, however, the parking lot was filled with the wrecked cars of the residents—with dents, and different colored fenders, and smashed windows, and bumpers falling off.

At the bus stop on my way to work the first morning, I met one of my neighbors, who had recently been released from prison.

"The criminal courts," he said, "describe me as an 'habitual offender.' The ground-level apartment the manager offered you previously had a 'nice' guy living there, who shot his girlfriend in the head five times, with her father just outside the door. It was on the news and everything."

I was relieved that I had chosen an apartment where no one had been killed recently.

When I had lived in Pennsylvania seven years earlier, the ghettos didn't look like paradise, the way they do in Florida, so I had just unwittingly moved into one of the worst neighborhoods in town. If I had a death wish, all I had to do was walk 200 feet down the street at night, and I would almost certainly get shot. Also, many of the other apartment buildings were "decorated" with broken blinds and pinned-up sheets over the windows. I didn't like coming home to this depressing environment after work.

To top it off, the night security guard looked so high that it made me wonder if he would assist a robber in holding me up. At the same time, I was empathetically overwhelmed by the thought of the problems he had doing security work in one of the worst parts of town. No wonder I saw so much suffering in his dark glassy eyes.

(Play "Hard Love," by Need to Breathe.)

All I could do was decide to see the bright side of the situation. For the amount of money I was spending, my apartment was nice and roomy. And again, one of my life's greatest spiritual moments came from living in this situation.

I tried to stop fearing God enough to channel Him, because at that point I needed the universe's highest being onboard with me. I was upset about everything I was going through and wanted His explanation for it. *Was all this happening to bring me closer to Him?* Some of the most amazing things happened through those experiences.

First, I will say that, at that time in my life, in an

attempt to be honest, I had a way of expressing myself with curse words. In the heat of the moment, I asked God, "Did You ever beat the shit out of me to teach me something?"

God replied in a *very* heartfelt way, "No."

When I had channeled in the past, the divine voice sounded the same as my thoughts. However, at this point in my channeling, I was starting to distinguish between God's voice and my own. God's expressions, unlike mine, were continuously loving. He didn't take offense at my curse words. I didn't mean anything by them, anyway. His *no* was actually a loving reply.

I started to realize that the God I was learning about through experience did not seem to be at all revengeful. So, I went on a personal quest, asking random people about their relationship with God. Although they all had a non-channeling relationship with God, they said that He was a loving God. This was the beginning of an amazing awakening for me.

As I continued to meditate, I asked God why I was going through so many hardships, and He said the most amazing thing, "To make you worthy of your fame."

WHAT!? I thought. *I'm becoming famous???*

"How?" I asked.

"The book you're writing is going to be made into a movie."

It became obvious to me that that would certainly open the door to fame. Nonetheless, when God told me about my future fame, I immediately started to reflect on everything I had been through. Everything difficult had begun to happen to me when I started asking for unlimited income. Perhaps the universe was somehow now answering my prayers. It seemed that my new life would bring a larger, renewed purpose that I didn't fully realize I had until I kept channeling God.

I remembered when Jess told me that part of my life's purpose, in addition to being a DJ, is to help people with their spiritual lives. When she told me that, she explained that spiritual people often go through a serious crisis before they can help others. Also, the bigger the person's purpose, the bigger his or her crisis. I also remembered from the Bible that God often chooses previously broken people like me to serve a greater purpose.

A schizophrenic with a spiritual purpose? I wondered.

Who is going to believe me?

(Play "Pink Houses," by John Mellencamp.)

However, God's amazing qualities did not stop there.

My leasing manager had never had the apartment cleaned, so it was infested with every bug in the state. Totally disgusting! Savannah hated coming over and seeing me living in that filth. You can imagine what it was like, not being able to prepare food on the counter because some creatures had been running around there a minute before.

The apartment had been vacant for three months prior to my moving in, so there was food left everywhere dehydrated from the heat. Although I was proud to be out of the shelter, that apartment was nearly impossible to live in. When I called the leasing manager about the bugs, she told me that the exterminators would be coming on Wednesday.

That Tuesday morning, when I found a million tiny white dots in the kitchen sink, I mentally asked God, *Did the white dots come from the bugs?*

"Yes," flashed gently in my mind in white letters as I heard His loving voice.

Should I kill the bugs?

"No."

Should I collect the eggs and put them outside?

"Yes."

I could feel the loving energy behind His words.

Did God have so much compassion for all His living creations that I should not exterminate them?

Although it was extremely painful for me, I chose to listen to God and didn't kill the bugs. I just knew in my heart that everything would be okay, so I said to God, *If you prevent the exterminators from showing up on Wednesday, I won't call the leasing office to bring the pest control people out here.*

When I called Savannah that night, she said, "I think you're completely nuts for leaving the bugs in your apartment."

Guess what? When that Wednesday came around, the exterminators magically never showed up! That's when something even more amazing happened. But first, so you will understand, let me do a little explaining.

At that time, it was getting harder and harder for me to show up at my sales job. Through spiritual wisdom, I learned that life becomes more difficult when you're doing something that is no longer your life's purpose. In other words, I knew that if my life were starting to suck, that was a sign from Heaven above that this sales job was not my life's purpose.

My time at my desk became a living hell. Somehow, *every* dead sales lead in the whole company came to me! Finally, in desperation, I channeled God quietly at my desk to see if I should leave the company.

The reply was clear and bold: "YES."

That was the loudest, clearest answer I ever got in my short history of channeling. God had made it super loud, knowing that I would have thought His response was nonsense if it were said calmly.

When I began to worry that I would have to put in two-weeks' notice, God said in a loving way, "Just leave."

So I stood up, put my headset down on the desk, and walked over to the supervisor with fearless confidence.

It was an indescribable pivotal moment when I said to him, "My poor sales were not caused by a lack of training on your part or insufficient performance on my part. I'm leaving the company because I know I have bigger things elsewhere. It's nothing personal."

The supervisor was really cool and didn't take offense.

God was right about walking out!

I didn't even need to give a two-weeks' notice! I was completely elated!

On my way home from work, I called Savannah, who thought I was completely crazy.

"If I live with you, and we start a family, you can't just go quitting your job one day because of a channeled answer. How are you going to pay for our apartment? You need a plan! When big responsibilities are in the picture, you need to have plans and work toward them! You can't just quit your job out of nowhere!"

But here's where the next miracle happened! My mom called the next day to tell me that my long-lost Puerto Rican step-family would probably be able to give me a place to stay. Because I hadn't spoken to them in many years, I never felt right about asking them to help me. Nonetheless, they welcomed me into their home with open arms. It was the most refreshing thing to realize that Hispanic cultures are often more family-oriented than Anglo ones. In fact, they were so loving and supportive that it was *extremely* refreshing. So, as it turned out, I didn't have to look for a place to stay because the place basically found me.

(Play "Eye of The Storm" (Featuring Gabe Real) by Ryan Stevenson.)

But then came an even bigger miracle.

I had been living in my apartment for a little too long to cancel the lease on account of buyer's remorse. But since I had listened to God and not killed the bugs, the leasing manager let me out of my lease for uninhabitable conditions. I realized that, whenever I had faith, I came out a winner. So, I moved in with my step-family and received my deposit back in the mail without a single question!

Now that I didn't have an apartment to pay for anymore, that was a big relief. It was then that I profoundly realized the value of God's simple masterful suggestions. Thinking back on it now, I was absolutely convinced that my imagination could never have construed such a plan during those channelings because I had no clue what God had in store for me next. All I had was faith and guidance.

Another New Life

When I moved in with my step-family, I felt that my loving ways had earned me this place to stay through the law of attraction, since I was continuously focusing on love in my spiritual life. God's blessings were also a part of the bigger plan.

My step-family set my rent at only $400 per month and gave me emotional support. Miraculously, they even made the family car available to me for my mobile DJ work.

During this period, I listed myself on two prominent booking sites for high-energy, mainstream DJ'ing. Between the two sites, I soon accumulated twenty-three five-star reviews for my talent. I loved having people rave about my performances.

I felt that the Divine was helping to move me away from being in sales by giving me the means necessary to carry out my life purpose as a DJ. My great new diverse DJ experience came about when I got booked for a wide variety of crowds and occasions.

You're Unlimited

In these spiritual wisdom books, I learned that the higher self is the part of you that also exists in a realm where all beings share a consciousness.[12] It is the combination of your soul and your spirit. If you meditate on positive qualities that you want, your higher self can give you an endless supply of them. For example, your higher self can give you an endless supply of love for yourself and patience for other people, and you can tap into those qualities whenever you wish. It can also give you an endless supply of confidence and fearlessness.

Our higher self is the midpoint between us and our inner fragment of God. It knows what God knows, including our future; and although we forgot this when we were born, we are capable of remembering that there's an *endless* supply of everything that's good already within us.

After I became familiar with my higher self through channeling, I began using that awareness to budget my

---

[12] Sanaya Roman, *Spiritual Growth: Being Your Higher Self* (Tiburon, CA: H. J. Kramer Inc, 1989).

money and found that it worked perfectly. My imagination can't predict my finances but my higher self definitely can!

If I channel my higher self and mentally ask, *Do I have money for* . . . and get an immediate response, such as a voice or impulse, I disregard it, because although the ego wants to protect you through fear, it's probably answering for my higher self, and the ego is pretty much wrong one hundred percent of the time.[13] I believe that emotional fear is a lie attempting to be truth. So, when this happens, I wait for the slower sensation in the body or a message that comes to me. For me, these messages from my higher self were internal sensations—more specifically, discomforts residing in the body.

---

[13] Virtue, *Angel Therapy.*

Why We Need a Control & Protection

Since there are things in the spiritual dimension that can play pranks on your channeled messages, again it's good to pray to and focus solely on God so that your messages are purely from Him. In spirituality, a control is a divine being that makes sure your psychic channeling is going to your intended recipient, and is being protected.

If for example, if you choose to channel your guardian angel, a divine control would make sure there is no interference between you and your guardian angel. Therefore, according to the will of God and your control, the message would be protected against interference from lower beings or prank-spirits. It has been said, once you start a regular practice of channeling, a control may come to you and ask if it can assist you. However, I found that God is the ultimate control and source.

When God teaches you to discern the false messages of darkness from the loving truthful messages of the light, He may allow interference to happen during your channeling, so that you learn experientially the difference between the two sources. So it's good to use common sense, or better yet, your sixth sense, when receiving any information from the spirit realm. You can always turn inward for answers, because you should already know in your loving heart what the answer should be.

Always stay connected to the emotional sensations in your body, along with any intuitive information. If something does not resonate with your heart and these internal guides you should not listen to, or follow through with it. After all, God is continuously speaking to you through your internal feelings about a situation. As long as you always stay focused on the light, the darkness will always be limited as much as possible.

Reading Savannah's Mind

During my stay at my grandmother's, she eventually developed affection for Savannah and allowed her to go into my bedroom. As I lay in bed with my prized girlfriend, I was reading about basic telepathy in an Orin book, so I tried it out with Savannah.

I asked her to pick a number between one and 100. I closed my eyes and pretended I was her as she was choosing her number. After a moment, a number flashed into my mind in white letters. I said,

"52?"

"What????" she yelled.

She started crying, saying she was scared by it. I realized telepathy is really a possibility and empathically calmed her down.

It's worth noting here that I could only channel information from Savannah's mind that her higher self would allow me to have. It is known in spirituality that psychics can receive information from another person's aura but only to the degree that their higher self permits the channeler to have. This is commonly said to be true for everyone. Also, from my experience, when the Divine has sent previously unknown information to psychics, it has always been for the highest good of those involved.

New Rainbows

Savannah and I were beginning to awaken to the magic of the universe. On our way to the beach one day, we felt drawn to the metaphysical store. After we entered the store, she felt immediately drawn to a particular stone.

"What's this?" she asked the store's guru.

"It's rainbow quartz. See how it sort of has a rainbow in it?"

"Oh wow!" she said.

"It stands for new beginnings."

Already feeling this could make a heartfelt gift, I purchased one for Savannah and myself.

We arrived at the beach and floated our blankets onto the sand. I lay down with my eyes closed next to Savannah and took in all the healing energy from around me.

"Look! How incredible!" she said.

"Oh my gosh!" I said.

When I opened my eyes, there was a rainbow right in our line of vision, and there hadn't been any sign of rain.

We took the rainbow in the sky as a sign of new beginnings, ironically almost immediately after being drawn to purchase a rainbow quartz crystal. The universe had begun to work in magical, synchronistic ways.

This divine "technology" is majestically beautiful.

Higher Self -Heart/Mind

At this point, I had been reading literature, dieting as a vegan, affirming, praying, and doing everything I could to increase my psychic abilities. I wanted to be a better channel so that I could receive divine guidance to help me with my life.

Dieting is well known to facilitate channeling and psychic abilities. Vegans frequently believe that there is negative energy in most meat because the animal was suffering right before it was killed. Consuming this negative energy can psychically block you from the spiritual dimension. There is also negative energy in dairy products, too, which vegans avoid for the same reason.

Higher, loving energy is essential in communicating with and attracting loving divine beings into your presence through God's law of attraction. Therefore vegans often eat a plant-based diet to facilitate psychic connections with the Divine.

For the previous three years, I had adopted all these measures intensively to increase my connection with my divine support team. I also began drinking Synergy raw kombucha drinks, about once every day. I noticed they started to make me very receptive to psychic abilities.

Because of all my dieting, one day a voice began speaking in my mind continuously. It was slightly louder than my ordinary thinking, saying, "Yes . . . No . . . Yes," in response to every thought I had. I was wise enough to question this voice. I mentally asked, *Where do you come from?*

It said, "The self."

I thought, *The personality self . . . the ego self?*

It said, "The higher."

I was completely floored because I knew this is a part of my being that was unlimited!

Over the next few days, my higher self reintroduced me to the way it communicates to me through what is also known as my "heart/mind." For example, if I'm on the wrong pathway in my life it sends a pain through my heart center. When I'm on the right path there's a good sensation in my heart. If it wants me to stop and channel it, it will send an enormous pain somewhere in my body that won't go away until I stop and channel it. If it doesn't want me to merge right on the highway it will send a pain somewhere on the right side of my body right before I'm about to merge. I will recheck my mirrors and notice there is something in the way of shifting lanes.

After the higher self introduced me to the way it communicates with me through my body, its voice disappeared, and I was left sensing this newly relearned communication of pain/love bodily sensations.

I still wanted additional psychic abilities, so I kept praying for them. I admit that I was afraid to make decisions on my own because, after all I had been through, I didn't want to make a wrong decision in life that would lead to more suffering. I tried going through my higher self for every decision. When I did that it started leading me down the wrong paths for making me stand on my own two feet.

Once my higher self led me down the "wrong" path, I asked my spirit guides, and my spirit guides led me down the "wrong" path, and then I asked God, and God led me down the "wrong" path, as well. There was no one to turn to besides my own love integrity.

In the previous paragraph, "wrong" is a misnomer,

because "wrong" is based on societies' common beliefs, not God's. A full attempt at explaining my perception of God's perception was beyond my comprehension of Him at this point in my channeling. However, I hope to advance my readers to the point of understanding my experience with God's ways in future books.

Nonetheless, the reader should note that although there is an unlimited amount of heavenly support, you can't ask the Divine for every single answer in life; otherwise, you're not living your own life. These resources want you to stand on your own two feet and in your own power and take responsibility for your decisions. The light will teach you to think for yourself and teach you loving ways that come from your heart. The Divine had future plans for my learning, but the first step was to teach me an evolved way of living, and those answers came from the heart.

These communications and what I began learning taught me how to be "sensitive" and intuitive. It's like an art of balance. As I received channeled information, I had to discern if it came from the light. The information could be abstract, challenging, and surprisingly correct; however, one misplaced decision while following this guidance could also leave you with a setback or a lesson to learn.

As I sensed my way through things, I learned to think for myself and listen to what I sensed was correct, disregarding what I sensed could be wrong. But at first I was "young" in my learning this.

A recurring theme in this book is that if you're ever in a position where you have no heavily resources, you can let wise love guide you and you will make better decisions that way. All one needs is just a little bit of wise love.

Higher Self Prevents a Low Situation

For some reason, my higher self was guiding me, through sensations in my body, not to buy some really inexpensive items I knew that I could afford. This series of events caused me to leave Walmart early just to land me in a situation while walking out.

A man in a van was driving by and yelling at Savannah as if he didn't know his boundaries with women. He saw me quickly walking toward her and left. Savannah was praying that I would appear there to help her.

Thank God my higher self won the situation and got me out of the store to deter anything potential from happening. As I comforted Savannah, I realized that the spiritual dimension can work in mysteries that can be confusing until you see the larger scheme of things. The higher self and God see a bigger plan than we can, and they are there to protect and enlighten us, especially when we stay focused on them, which attracts their presence.

World Peace

In God's divine timing, He answered my prayer by giving me "psychic abilities" and signs that were so strong I would not have ever predicted they would appear in such abundance. These experiences can't easily be explained with words. All I can say is that at this stage there were signs from God everywhere, outside of my body, that go perfectly along with everything that I am thinking in the very moment, which truly never happened before. Therefore, unless everything I experienced externally was entirely a hallucination, I can't deny that God was communicating with me whenever He wanted to say something.

For example, I began wanting my book to influence world peace, so I asked God to help me. I was in Walgreens that night, thinking about this, and when I looked up, right in front of me during at that exact moment was a magazine title that said "World Peace Starts Here." Then I looked to my side and someone just standing there talking to someone else pointed at a TV in front of us, and as I drew my attention to it, the commercial literally started to gracefully say in perfect timing, “I will take you there.”

How did that just happen? I wondered.

Immediately after that, I looked to the person who was standing next to the person who pointed, and she said, in perfect timing,

“Isn’t this a wonderful thing?”

The person she was speaking with said, “Yeah it really is. I can help you with that anytime you ask for it.”

I walked out of Walgreens thinking *God is with me.* In perfect timing a gentle alert went off over the intercom, as if it in perfect timing, which gave me the feeling that He was replying to me in some perfectly mysterious way that I can’t easily explain, saying “Yes.”

I knew something mysterious, boundless, and gracefully perfect was there. Something completely limitless. Something that could read my mind and use anything as a means of communicating with me, externally, as if it already had a divine plan in place to answer my thoughts. As I walked out of the store in a deep state of connection I thought, *God might help me.* I slowed down looking for a response and literally, in perfect timing, the exit door opened, as if it were personified and saying, “Yes sir, I am helping you, right this way please.”

It was an indescribable state of constant connection.

I continued to get more signs as I left the store. I began to wonder if Jesus was helping me, too. In the parking lot, as I was backing my car out of the parking space, with impeccable timing, right in front of me was a bumper sticker that said, “Jesus loves you.”

What? I thought, *how did that get there in perfect timing with my thought?*

Then as I continued backing out of the space, I turned around, looked behind me with my window down, and a woman walking by me, in miracle timing, said to someone, “Yeah, isn’t that great, he’s everywhere, isn’t he?”

There were even more signs when it actually happened, but this is the basic model of how God communicates with me through constant external signs and people. I was learning from experience that God’s mysterious, yet unmistakable communications comes literally through every outlet He decides to use. I can only describe it is a beautiful, limitless, and loving magic that’s completely beyond any words. It is a genteelly instant contact that is completely synchronistic and loving, whenever you listen for it and absolutely believe it's there.

When God sent me the first signs, they were also accompanied by a subtle electric-like sensation in my body that caused an elevated awareness. Again, to me, there was absolutely no mistaking that God was there speaking through signs and people. Where there used to be randomness in the background around me, there was now mysterious contact though God who spoke a language that was directly in response to my thinking and listening.

I have been receiving signs like this all day every day, practically since it began. Whenever I ask God a question, there's almost always an immediate yes or no right in front of me. It's direct enough to understand yet mysterious enough to require me to have to believe in it for it to work. Let me explain to the reader that I'm well enough to have my bearings in reality and to know this is not a trillion-series of grand coincidences or a symptom of schizophrenia. I now know the difference through experience, and for you to experience this too if you wish, you will have to just believe, let go, allow, listen, and discern if it is from the light or not.

I also learned that I could detach myself from divine communication by taking a step back and not listening to it from time to time, to maintain a sane balance. It took me some adjusting to get used to it, but eventually there was so much love that it became a part of my life that I never wanted to do without.

I began sharing these spiritual experiences with a nonjudgmental, online spiritual community. One member reported back to me that she had very similar spiritual experiences with God. Many of the regular people, apparently non-schizophrenic and healthy, on that webpage were reporting evolved metaphysical and psychic experiences. And when I went to a metaphysical store, I spoke with other psychics who knew things about me that only I knew.

My point is that it wasn't just me or only schizophrenics who have similar experiences. If you followed my footsteps for divine communication, any open-minded person would eventually become aware and see the truth, unless they were in a state of crippling denial or disbelief, in which case such a state would attract circumstances that would cause the person to disbelieve anyway.

During this time, God's signs were an outright display of his graceful, yet unlimited power to do absolutely anything. As these things were happening to me, I kept mentally asking the angels over and over, *All things are possible through God, right?*

Every single time I asked that question, I saw a flash of white light that indicated my guardian angel was lighting a loving "Yes!"

Once a continuous stream of communication was established, God asked me, "What do you want for Christmas?"

I said mentally, *To be with my girlfriend . . . world peace . . . for everyone to have their dreams come true and to have Earth's inhabitants set free from limitation.*

The reader may notice that my Christmas gift was mainly gifts to the world. God responded to this thought many times by saying that this is possible, but we also have dues to pay on this Earth; because of this, life can't be perfect. I believe God was talking about how He sometimes uses the darkness to bring us to the light.[14] He

---

[14]Neale Donald Walsch, *Conversations with God: an uncommon*

led me to understand that everything needs balance to work properly.

After receiving that message, I began to stop taking my medicine for schizophrenia. The doctor I was working with actually encouraged this, saying that I was doing so well that we could slowly decrease the medicine to see how I am doing.

God, the angels, my spirit guides, and my higher self all seemed to guide me in this direction, so I stopped my medication.

After a few weeks or so, this loud, booming, and controlling voice came over me claiming to be God. It started commanding things to me. It basically said, "I am the God of all Gods. I created everything in your existence. I will completely destroy you, your entire family, and everything in your existence unless you make a commitment to me, in order to receive what you want for Christmas."

By this point, I had witnessed a million small miracles from God and was not about to mess with Him, based on my fears about Him from the Bible. I also knew at some

---

dialogue (New York, NY: G.P. Putnam's Sons, 1995).

level that there was nothing He couldn't save me from. Since I didn't take my medicine, I unknowingly started to become mentally handicapped again. I also didn't have the discernment to realize that this message wasn't from the loving God I knew all along.

The booming voice then told me to set the house on fire. In my defense, I was mentally handicapped and no one was home with me, and so, fearing this commanding entity, I set a small area of the kitchen floor on fire with a little bit of gasoline. I drove to the store and came back to see that there was only a black spot on the tile floor and that nothing in the home was really damaged.

Ironically, the pastor of the church pulled into the driveway to drop off Samantha and told me to call the cops. The cops came, and this so-called "God" led me to lie to them. Needless to say, when my brother heard I set the kitchen on fire, he committed me to a mental institution so I could become stabilized on medication again.

The police found me that night in my car when this aggressive, abusive voice pushed me to stay parked next to a guardhouse at a gated community entrance.

After I was released from the hospital, medicated and

stabilized, I mentally asked God, *"Was that you?"* [The night of the booming voice.] Something from the spirit realm said, "It was a demon."

I thought, *Did that happen because I stopped taking my medicine (and became vulnerable to a demon attack?)*

God said, "Yes, and it will happen again if you don't take your medicine."

Interestingly enough, God went on to say in a caring, genuine way, "Even if *I* tell you to do something [destructive] like that you shouldn't listen."

I thought that God had a very loving, humble response. That was the God I was used to hearing, and it resonated with my inner being.

The next day, I went to my spiritual community and found that, at the same time this happened to me, a lot my fellow spiritual people were miraculously experiencing similar problems with demons coming through on their communications. I explained what happened to me, and an experienced psychic replied to my thread saying, "God was orchestrating, through all of us, what is called a 'test of discernment.'"

Looking back on this, I feel that God was evolving my

channeling to help me discern what I am channeling, to listen to my heart before following through with any plans from the spiritual dimension, and to take my medicine, even if God told me not to! I realized that, all along, God was super loving and always worked with my own will or desire to create good. Conversely, it was the demon that was attacking, aggressive, abusive, and working against my own will to carry out lower acts or behaviors. Boy, how humiliating it was to have been fooled—and thank God for the care and light to clearly glean the difference.

As I reflected on this situation, it got me thinking about how close I was to the spiritual dimension I was when I was off my medication, yet how I couldn't process what was happening enough to understand that I was doing the wrong thing by listening to it.

God

After I was medicated for a short while and feeling mentally clear again, God wanted me to explain about how all of us will have to pay some type of dues on Earth, which I believe are part of bringing us back to the light. If you have health problems, spirituality can greatly reduce suffering but the inevitable is that you can't completely eliminate all of your suffering all of the time.

Since there is good and evil on Earth, there must be some type of suffering for some type of good to happen, so that we remember how great we are after we overcome the darkness.[15]

God has a way of seeing everything as "good," because, without the "bad" there can be no way to measure our greatness. Therefore, God's darkness is only there for higher things to happen.[16] An awakened being remembers that the highest truth is love; therefore, when we *are* love, we are truth. To stay in constant awareness that we are

---

[15] Walsch, *Conversations with God.*
[16] Walsch, *Conversations with God.*

love, that we are our highest qualities, and we are all connected, I believe is a level of evolution and part of a spiritual awakening.

I realized that, like the angels, God can send signs through music, commercials or TV dialog, as well. (I want the reader to note here that there have also been hundreds of cases where scientists set out to disprove paranormal phenomena but concluded there was more than meets the eye regarding metaphysical spirituality.[17])

I started to interpret the divine messages I was receiving through music. During the occasion I describe below, when I thought of the points God was making to me while listening to the song, the angels would also appear as dots and flashes of light, to confirm whether I had the correct idea. This seemed to be the way in which God was training me on how to spiritually receive messages through music.

The message below was written right after my channeling and prayer for the angels to assist me in remembering what happened during those channelings. It has been edited slightly for clarity:

---

[17] Roman and Packer, *Opening to Channel.*

This message started when the spiritual dimension led me in different directions, which helped me to stand on my own two feet regarding discernment, and as a result, caused my relationship with God to weaken. The angels also gave me several angel numbers that, when I looked them up during this channeling session, caused me to realize that I needed to strengthen my relationship with God. It was a little intimidating after the whole demon experience, but I had enough faith in the Divine to agree.

I will start by saying that I don't want the reader to hang on my every word like a lawyer, because the messages that God gave me came through music, in perfect timing with my thoughts, and were not the exact intention of the song lyrics according to the artist's original expression. In other words, it was about what the lyrics meant to me in the moment I was channeling God, not what the song actually meant.

During these experiences, certain lyrics came in perfectly timed response to questions I asked God, and when I heard the lyrics, they resonated with so that I knew which lyrics to listen to and what not to listen to. This became the model for everyday music channelings.

At first, I was guided to be honest with God. He told me He was "titanium" and nothing I said could bring Him down. I told Him about my relationship difficulties with Him, and then listened for His response. I thought I needed to drive to listen to the radio, but He communicated that He didn't want me driving long distances, and then I realized I was very low on gas money. So, I only drove to the nearby store for my grandmother's soda and then realized I had no wallet on me. During that trip, He literally said he was a mystery. I thought about it and this was right. His ways and communications have been mysterious since the dream I had during my stay with Jess. Then He said He's always watching me and knows my every move. He knew that that would make me worry a little, so He and the angels said not to worry though an angel number through observing the time on the clock.

I got home and He guided me to play my Calvin Harris station on iHeart radio. I turned it on and iHeart automatically started building and playing that station, which I never remember listening to previously. (It usually took me back to the station I listened to last, but this time it went straight to Calvin Harris's artist station.) God was using that moment's style of music to speak to me, and I was flattered. He told me, "Don't you worry child" [Heaven's got a plan for you], and I assumed it meant fame and fortune. After several songs, I felt my relationship and trust in God improving markedly. I asked for clarity about what I should play as a DJ, because I wanted to be a positive leader in my own way. He told me to play whatever I wanted and it wouldn't matter to Him, but if I appealed to darkness, I'd be "dancing with a 'friendly' devil [dark entities]." Feeling stronger in my relationship with God, I told him that I thought I needed some way to bring people closer to Him. I then made the point to Him that it's impossible for me to be perfect with music lyrics, because I was a mainstream DJ and mainstream music with less darkness is rare. (Aside from this channeling, I want to encourage more artists to consciously create music with messages that are higher, to work with the law of attraction and bring good things into the listener's life.)

He then told me that our relationships with Him are, to a degree, dysfunctional or crazy. He builds us up, He tears us down, He keeps us guessing, and everything in between. He said He is always close to us and we can always turn back to Him for strength and support. He will be our "clarity."

I realized that because of this process we'll always have to renew our relationship with God and the Divine continuously over our lifetimes. He told me that I would never know if He would maintain my wealth and fame for the rest of my life, but I have to take that road and basically brave it with Him. He mentioned that as long as I am faithful, I will have my girlfriend, Savannah and that she was a gift to me from Heaven.

At some point, He mentioned something to me about world peace, because I wanted this book to influence it. He told me that the world will always be uncertain and that it was His job to work with that. He said that it's our work to find our own inner peace in ourselves despite any of the world's uncertainty. (Therefore, world peace was about a journey of inner peace.)

I was afraid of receiving an intrusive message from a demon, but when I looked at the clock in that exact moment, the angel number I received from it told me to release my fears to the Divine and keep positive thoughts, so I did. I also worried about the channeling going all night like it did when I was off my medication.

I believe that since I kept positive thoughts everything worked out with my divine communication. God reminded me that if I kept channeling that night and stayed in His peaceful presence I would be avoiding going to bed. So, I chose to stop the channeling and went to sleep.

That concluded my channeling.

If you think about it, uncertainty is just a part of life. I believe that God wants us to find inner peace in our life's uncertainty the same way he wants us to find inner peace amid the world's uncertainty. I will mention repeatedly that it takes faith and thoughts of love to bring us through uncertainty without worry. We are surrounded by heavenly beings who won't let us die before our time, and they are always working for us. Everything happens for a reason, and through God, I know that all things are possible.

One thing I learned from my schizophrenic episode is that I should try to balance my life. I find that being over serious and unloving about anything can lead anyone to darkness.

For example, when we work too much, the unbalance can affect our health. Metaphorically speaking, we can be plagued with the demons of not eating healthy if we make the wrong food choices. Sometimes we are affected by the metaphoric demons of not seeing our family. However, if we have too much family in our life, our job could suffer.

When spending is out of balance it could affect our work habits, and so on—we need balance in everything we do.

God wants you to know that sometimes "bad" things have to happen for "good" things to happen. I believe this is why darkness can happen to "good" people, as well. When we have reached mastery, we will make the best of our suffering, knowing we will overcome it through the loving God within.

My current Earthly aim is to stay in Heaven after I pass, among the ascended masters who make continuous and loving contributions to Earth from Heaven's vantage point, because the life of the soul never dies. I believe that when we "die," we help out our Earthly brothers and sisters even more than we did while we were alive.

Who Am I?

I couldn't help but ask a curious question: *If I was making contact with God, does that make me a prophet? Does that make other people who have done so prophets?* It occurred to me that anyone could be a prophet if they wanted to make contact with God; however, when I walked by the TV thinking of this, the TV literally and directly said, "You are not a prophet" in the dialog of the show that was on. I took this as a very clear sign that I'm not. However, after much contemplation, I was never completely sure if this message came from the light or not, so it remained a little mysterious to me.

After this happened, in the back of my mind, I felt that past lifetimes are real and I wondered who I may have been previously. *Who was I?*

A Beautiful Plan

At this juncture, I was still living with a roommate, Samantha, at my grandmother's. Although she was extremely religious, I sensed that Samantha had her own psychic abilities, because she told people things she heard God say while she was praying.

One delightful evening I was sitting with my stepmom and Samantha.

"God has something beautiful planned for you. I don't know exactly what it is, but it's going to be incredible!" Samantha said to me.

Hmmm, I thought with a smile, *this is ironic, because she has absolutely no idea I'm writing this book that God is indicating will be a success.*

Affirmation and Manifestation

For those who believe in the law of attraction, your thoughts become prayers that allow you to attract many of the circumstances you think about. These situations will be higher or lower, simply by virtue of what you spend time thinking about. For example, as you are aware, I stayed focused on love and appreciation in my spiritual life, and that manifested into a loving place for me to stay with my step-family, because I believed it would.

As you know, there was a time in my life where God didn't answer a single prayer of mine and I started to wonder if he was listening or even existed out there anywhere. After I developed spiritually, I discovered that all prayers are answered; however, it's up to God's will to provide these answers to you in a way that serves your soul, or higher good. Since God wants our successes to serve our soul in the best way possible, and since I believed I would be spiritually prepared before I received my gifts, I needed to learn how to figure out what God was trying to teach through my setbacks.

These setbacks helped me learn to reflect on life during meditative activities and helped me in the ways that I wanted to grow before publishing this book. The key to unlocking such growth lessons is to see the grander picture of things, which is discussed in more depth later on in this book.

Answers to prayers and affirmations also come according to divine timing, and as I desired to grow, my ability to co-create with God by using the law of attraction became stronger. I eventually began to see the circumstances some thoughts created on an everyday level. I did my best to create with it—among other things, world peace, an easy work life, and a better life for others in the community. I also began to make contact with more and more spiritual people, which gave me some opportunity to give guidance to them.

When I shared that I was writing a book about helping schizophrenia with spiritual principles, I immediately started finding and reaching people who wanted to heal themselves and guide other schizophrenics.

I found that many people, even some who are scientifically minded, believe that humans are evolving right now. Much of this evolution is happening spiritually and through psychic senses that allow everyday people to receive heavenly guidance. People everywhere are starting to find more peace, balance, healing, and love bestowed from the spiritual dimension but don't speak of it. Again, they don't want to be judged by others who aren't experienced with this topic.

I ask the reader to please not make assumptions or value-based judgments about this without having experience of it. I also found evolution doesn't happen to you unless you invite and manifest it in your life, sometimes over a period of years.

For any scientific-minded individuals who may want to prove this phenomenon, I feel that if one were able to track God's light, then perhaps empirical evidence of channeling could be obtained, since light enters the body when a divine message is received.[18]

I want the reader to make the best of their life, too. So, the remainder of this book is devoted to spiritual and self-improvement principles, schizophrenia as it relates to

---

[18] Roman and Packer, *Opening to Channel.*

spirituality, and some divine spiritual teachings, as well.

High Powers

First, I want to redefine for the world what Earthly power really is, and then I will teach you how to get anything according to your and God's will in your Earthly lifetime. In my younger years, I always wondered what power really is. My thoughts were polluted by the media into a thoughtform of a powerfully corrupt person doing harmful things to people through fear or drama. As I grew and spiritually developed, I learned a lot about power through the eyes of silent observation. After reflecting on what I observed, I can tell you what divine power is and how to get it.

Many people will agree that God is the ultimate power in the universe. But for a moment, let's pretend that God doesn't exist. Let's pretend that everything in the divine cosmic conscious doesn't exist. In other words, there are no angels, no gods or goddesses, and no ascended masters. At this point, I would say that the highest power in such a universe is love. God made love the highest power in our Earthly universe. He had to make evil in this existence because evil exists when people have *full* freedom of choice. However, I believe that love rules over evil in every universe God created.

My first step in increasing love is to increase your self-love. To love oneself is to make possible love to others. Loving oneself doesn't have to involve money, nor does it mean external perfection. Like peace, self-love starts with an inner journey. Then, once you have mastered self-love, you can move on to loving your outer world.

Sanaya Roman writes in *Living with Joy,* "You can help transform the planet. It does not take that many people focused on love to change the destiny of mankind, for love is one of the most powerful energies of the universe. It is thousands of times stronger than anger, resentment, or fear."[19]

I believe that if you want to perform a miracle without asking God to help, the highest power you could use to perform the miracle is love from the heart. A little bit of love can make anything work. Leading with love can solve

---

[19] Roman, *Living with Joy: Keys to Personal Power and Spiritual Transformation*
(Tiburon, CA: H. J. Kramer, 1986), p. 88.

problems because love is the highest truth. Love can bring together anything and make anything work, and with the absence of love, anything can be a failure.

If you remember any wrong you ever felt or experienced in a relationship, it can all be traced back to a lack of love in that situation. Love is strength, and many people have the wrong idea of strength. Strength is not fighting everything out with people. Strength can be redefined as rising above adversity to use love in your situation. We continuously need to remember that we are love, so that we may reach our own level of greatness.

When light is used in combination with love, it is even more powerful. For example, if you want to spiritually help heal something, even a situation, you can send it both light and love. To do this, it helps to know that light responds to your imagination. So, if you imagine it everywhere, it will be where you imagined it, in the fourth dimension.[20]

I must say that if you're planning to "use" love for the sake of having corrupt power or to manipulate people, you have the wrong intentions. It simply will not work, because

---

[20] Roman, *Spiritual Growth.*

intuitive people can sense sincerity.

Love is pure, free, open. Love from the heart has only higher intentions, and *wise* love wants only to carry out higher decisions. I have found through experience that the God of our universe and His angels teach us with wise love.

I observed from the spirit realm somehow that we have mastery if we continuously exist in love. To do this we must have high *self*-love.

Conversely, if someone is getting under your skin and loving them doesn't work, you need to love yourself enough to do something about it. Separating yourself from someone can be helpful until, after some time, you are ready to heal things with that person.

In a dispute, if you let love guide your actions, you can work something out or let it go without getting into a fight and making things worse, because again, love is freedom for the other person as well. In other words, love will set others free if a situation no longer serves you.

(Play "Power of Love" by Huey Lewis and the News.)

Master Teaching

In the Earth Life series by Orin and Sanaya Roman, Orin—a high-level spirit guide of light—explains what a master teacher is. He mentions that a master teacher never takes a learning experience away from someone and never does the work for them.

Jess was a teacher who taught children in a poverty-stricken neighborhood. They were raised in situations where the parents neglected the child's schooling, and she made them the most educated children in the whole school by the time she was done teaching them at the end of the year. She explained to me her master teaching secret: "Most parents take the project from the child and do it for them, for the sake of showing the child how to do it," said Jess. "Doing so has actually excluded the child of a learning experience."

Jess got her children to learn by letting them mess up the project on their own. Once they'd messed it up many times, they began to learn through trial and error, and they actually learned quicker in the long run. The teachers who picked up the projects and showed the children how to do them had the students with the least progress by the end of the year.

A master teacher can let someone make a mistake, or let them fail on their own in some instances, for the purpose of letting them learn a better way.

By all means, showing someone a higher way to do something from the start is good guidance, but if they are stubborn and insist on doing it their way, sometimes letting them learn the hard way will be their best teacher.

God, spirit guides, and angels could all teach you to learn something by guiding you in different directions. If they do, it will cause you to figure things out for yourself. I think that God created demons that get us going in the wrong direction so that it would eventually bring us back to Him, His love, and loving teachings in a grander scheme. Hopefully, this could teach us to learn to trust in Him and in doing things in His loving way.

Most importantly, Orin also explains that you should teach at the student's level, and at the rate they are able to learn. It is appropriate to teach the right step at each time. If someone can't handle the next step, then the teacher should wait until it is the right time or moment to teach that step. I believe it is important for a teacher to work with patient timing in the same way God teaches, through patient, graceful, divine timing.

The Law of Attraction

God created the law of attraction for ours and other universes. There are many laws that govern our existence, such as the law of increase and the law of pure potentiality. Some of these are mentioned in Deepak Chopra's book, *The Seven Spiritual Laws of Success*. But for now, I will focus on the law of attraction, specifically.

The law of attraction is a general secret that people need to have more awareness of. You are a co-creator with God and the beings that comprise our universe. Although you can't ultimately control every single thing with the law of attraction, you can still influence your future and the circumstances of it. This law is a beautiful thing that can be used to promote the greater good.

It is also worth noting that some believe you can co-create anything God wills for you, while others believe that you can receive only what is rightfully yours in your lifetime. It has been said that *we* allowed ourselves a certain amount and type of success in our life contract before we incarnated. Those who believe that commonly say our potential success is written in the Akashic record in Heaven. There are meditations one can do to access this record, but guiding you in that meditation is beyond the scope of this introductory spiritual book.

In order to get anything that is in God's will for you, as a good practice you should mentally say whenever you ask for something, " . . . *with harm to no one*." This way, it doesn't create the potential for a lower situation to happen while bringing what you have asked for. Furthermore, when you co-create with God, He will usually use divine timing to answer this "prayer."

I had a funny experience once with God, when I was wanting Him to hurry up and He said jokingly, "I don't tell you to hurry up do I?"

Another thing I will teach you about getting what you want out of life is that, again, all your thoughts act as prayers. All your thoughts are projected into your future to attract the situations and things you think about.[21] If you think about negative things, negative things will influence your future. If you think about positive things, positive

---

[21] Roman, *Spiritual Growth.*

things will influence your future. This also works more strongly with what you talk about.

For example, have you ever noticed how positive people seem to be blessed and have positive things happen to them more frequently? I believe this is because the law of attraction takes those thoughts, speech, and actions and helps to bring positive things into their future. If you don't have money, you may want to allow yourself to have it through positive thinking, speaking, and doing.

Also, it is common spiritual knowledge that the law of attraction exists in God's consciousness. God is so magical that He gives us all individual attention. He is constantly listening and creating with all of us on an individual level through our thoughts and prayers that immediately go into his consciousness when we think them.

It's good to know that fear is one of the most destructive emotions for people's lives and for the law of attraction. From a spiritual standpoint, when people don't have money it could be because they worry about bills and not having what they want. This worry uses the law of attraction to produce more situations that cause you to worry about what you want to have. Fear and lower energies can also attract can demons, and no one should invite them in so easily. A trick to getting more money without fearing is to spend what you have appropriately and not worry about or fear lack. Show the universe you genuinely appreciate and love what you already have.

There's a difference between the emotion of fear and being cautious. Caution in life is essential but the emotion of fear is not. Love is the opposite of fear and love is all there is, once we awaken to remember it.[22]

Emotions and beliefs will intensify the law of attraction. So, the object of the game is to make all of your thoughts, speech, emotions, beliefs, and actions positive so the law of attraction brings as many positive things as possible into your future. Again, please understand that there will be setbacks, even if you make every thought, spoken word, and action 100 percent positive. Learning about the process of creating what you want can create more happiness for you during times of suffering, since by thinking thoughts of happiness and well-being, you are creating those emotions. For more information on the law of attraction, see the recommended media section in the

[22] Walsch, *Conversations with God.*

back of this book.

If you catch yourself thinking a negative thought, let it go and instantly create a magical affirmation about what you do want. For example, if you start to worry about money, let it go and mentally affirm with good-mood energy, "Money is in endless supply for me." If you are suffering, magically affirm, *"I have found happiness."*

In regard to positive affirmations, Florence Scovel Shinn wrote a lot about a person's ability to manifest in magnificent ways. In *Your Word Is Your Wand,* she described one's language as being like a magic wand you can wave over a situation to remedy it.[23]

Viewing speech affirmations as magic is a very empowering way to view the strength of your words. As I have awakened more spiritually, I consciously remember the intent of her teachings, and I have frequently implemented them for effectiveness.

In addition, your vibration is something that influences what is magnetic to you through the law of attraction. Your vibration rate happens according to the type of energy in your body. When positive energy is in your body, your

---

[23] Virginia: Wilder Publications, 2009.

energy is vibrating at a higher level, you are a magnet to good circumstances, and you attract people with the same positive energy.

Thinking back in time, do you remember that when it rained, it poured? Remember when you were in a good mood and everything turned out your way? That's because your vibration made you a magnet to the circumstances you were in, as well as the type of people around you.

If you don't get what you're affirming right away, it's probably a good idea to consider asking God, or a psychic at a metaphysical store who has a desire to help the community and not just make money for clarity about your issue. In the beginning stages of my spiritual development, it took me from six months to over a year to attract some things that I affirmed every day. I even affirmed my fame for many years before it happened, knowing it was a part of my life purpose. Simply put, how fast the things that you affirm come to you can depend on how large of a request you are asking for, and how God's will is answering your request.

Some think your higher self knows what your future is and is always making sure you're experiencing the growth that you need for your future.[24] Take a moment and reflect on one of your life setbacks. Think about what you learned from the greater good in it, and how that wisdom helped you with your future. Your higher self or God had you learn that lesson so that you would be on track with your future path.

I think that if you're in a major setback the key is to not judge any of it as "bad." Look at the bigger picture to see how you can truly overcome your situation. That's what God created you for!

Another note about affirming is that you should be clear about what you want when you ask for it.[25] If you are flexible about how you receive what you want, it will come to you faster. So, for example, if you manifest a guitar by focusing on it, and are flexible enough to get a used or borrowed one, it could be created in your future faster.

Also, if you find that you don't get what you want soon enough, it is very important to have enough faith to carry

---

[24] Roman, *Living with Joy.*

[25] Sanaya Roman and Duane Packer, *Creating Money: Attracting Abundance*
(Tiburon, CA: H. J. Kramer/New World Library, 2007).

you all the way through, until you get what you're asking for. Some manifestations can come almost immediately and others take *years* to happen. When you see the reason why the manifestations are taking so long and you see the way you are being prepared to receive it, you'll appreciate the time it took because you'll see what you are getting is better than what you asked for.

I personally learned that correct timing was a large factor in bringing my manifestations faster into my life. We can't just "think" everything into existence, we need to also speak *and* take favorable action. Numerology and channeling help with knowing what step you're supposed to be taking in order to be aligned with the Divine in the timing of your manifestation.

When you begin to understand the law of attraction at much deeper levels, over a period of years, and you are focused on your skill at co-creating, your manifesting power can multiply. You will begin to take greater responsibility to think 100 percent positively and create a positive future for yourself and the world. However, if creating becomes too rapid when you can't think straight, you can always take a step back, so you are not in a more powerful creating mode—thus preventing a lower situation from manifesting.

The Cosmic Consciousness

In the spiritual dimension, there is a consciousness that's shared by all beings (God, angels, ascended masters, spirit guides, etc.). In this shared consciousness is the knowledge of everything that will ever be known about everything. This body of knowledge is commonly referred to as the universal mind or cosmic consciousness. It is God's consciousness. The universal mind is always listening to your thoughts and turning them into the physical reality that exists around you when it is in the manifestation cycle. As previously mentioned, the law of attraction is all in God's consciousness. All of your thoughts are heard in the cosmic consciousness, and all the beings in Heaven hear your every thought.

Like the Earthly seasons, manifestations happen in cycles, and it's good to know what part of this manifesting cycle you are in. Simply put, you are either in the positive thinking (prayer) stage, or you are in the letting go (and letting God) stage. Working with and receiving angel numbers and channeling God have been indicators for me to know when to stop affirming and let go in this cycle.

An interesting thing that God explained to me about cosmic consciousness is that it is possible for two different beings in Heaven to have access to all of God's knowledge and arrive at two different conclusions in response to the same question you may have. God and I both found this to be interesting.

At one point, my higher self was guiding me in one direction and God was guiding me in another. I asked God, *"How is it possible that both God and my higher self have access to the same information, yet both are guiding me in different directions?"*

God explained that He can see things my higher self can't, even though they both have the same body of knowledge. Yes, God can see things that other beings can't, even though they know the same thing. Interesting, right? God told me this when I mentally asked, and the song that was playing, appropriately, was, "I Can See for Miles" by The Who: "I [He] can see for miles, and miles, and miles."

Programming the Subconscious

You not only want to program the universal mind with positive thoughts and emotions, you also want to program your subconscious mind for good things.[26] Your subconscious mind does not know right from wrong. It is always listening to your thoughts and carrying them out as if they were orders. So, if you actually think to yourself, *"I'm so smart,"* you have just programed your subconscious mind and the neurons inside your mind to actually make you smart. Again, the key is to think, say, and try to believe good things. So, if you think empowering things over and over like, *"I'm a genius"* or *"I am the best of the best,"* you are programming your subconscious to be that, and you are using the law of attraction to co-create that into your reality. This is the basic framework on how you can begin to get or be anything great.

I program my subconscious knowing that all the cells in

---

[26]Florence Scovel Shinn, *The Magic Path of Intuition* (Carlsbad, California: Hay House, Inc., 2013).

my body are in communication with each other. This has been scientifically researched. You can literally tell your body things like, “I am not sick,” and it will program you to fight a virus. I use affirmations like this every time I feel a virus attacking my throat. I’ve never had a flu shot, and in an age of super viruses I almost never catch one because I mentally communicate positive things to my body and try to stay spiritually healthy. Typically, spiritually evolved people sense that spiritual health and physical health are nearly synonymous.

Affirmations are very powerful. With them, it has been said that you can limit aging, repair your body faster, and encourage your mind to overcome a mental health struggle.

Programming the subconscious and thinking empowering thoughts are things you want to remember in your darkest moments and toughest lessons. Positive thinking and healing are what got me through the most ridiculous life lessons. It is a *very* empowering way to live.

As you become better at manifesting, you will want to begin aligning yourself with people who think like you do and share common goals. When everyone shares a common goal, it will act like a chain prayer, as if everyone were praying for the same thing. If you can, you'll also want to surround yourself with people who have the same beliefs as you do.

The following meditation is similar to the Orin-life series meditations and others. I fully encourage you to take any spiritual knowledge you learn and comfortably modify it to what resonates with you. When you do this, you should follow your own higher guidance. After all, spiritual experience is different for each of us, and you want to practice it in a way that works best for you.

Meditation for Manifestation

If you start to meditate or channel, I recommend that you begin by first protecting yourself from the spiritual dimension. You can ask God or Archangel Michael to be present, protect you, and make sure your communications are happening with the beings you are intending to communicate with.

Another way to protect yourself, described in the book *Psychic Development for Beginners,* is to use your imagination to call light to your body and ask the light to always be there to protect you. The author also explains that you should meditate the next day, hold a picture of yourself in your mind during the meditation, and see if the light is still present around you when you see yourself. If it is not there in your mental picture, you need to keep programming the light until it automatically appears when you view a picture of yourself during your meditation. Michael, God, and the light are always near you when you concentrate on them, so you can be comfortable in your meditation space, knowing they are there.

Here are some simple steps to guide you if you would like to meditate for something you want.

1. Begin your meditation by lighting some incense, playing some meditation music, setting the mood for a peaceful meditation, and getting comfortable.

2. Close your eyes, take some deep breaths while focusing on your breathing, and just be. Take a moment to think some peaceful and calming thoughts that slow down your thinking.

3. Ask God to send you healing energy, noticing if you sense a positive shift of energy inside you when this happens.

4. Use your imagination to bring God's protective light around your body. Pack the light close to you so that it becomes concentrated and powerful.

5. Think of something you want in your life.

6. Imagine that you are attracting what you want by picturing each step in getting it and how good each step feels. Then, picture that what you want will come to you in a positive way.

7. Take another moment to just be, and open your eyes when you want to end the meditation.

8. Thank the universe for already bringing you what you want. Then, let go of what you are asking for so it is released into the universe.

(If you're serious about getting money or spiritual growth I highly recommend the books mentioned in the list of media at the end of this volume if you want to get more advanced meditations. Deepak Chopra's guided meditations are my recommended, masterful ways of awakening the infinite power that is already residing in your soul.)

In the following days, you should feel and think as if you have already manifested what you want.[27] Feel great and keep your vibration higher. Doing so will bring what you want to you faster. You should also give yourself positive affirmations like, "I love my new . . ." You should periodically repeat this meditation to make your affirmation/speech stronger, and also remember to let it go and let God create it when you get a divine sign that you are in that stage of the affirmation cycle. If a negative thought pops into your head, try backing it up with other positive thoughts of what you would actually want to

---

[27] Roman, *Spiritual Growth.*

happen.

For if you think a negative thought, it goes into a negative thought bin. Once the bin gets full the negative thoughts will actually come true. You want to fill that bin with positive thoughts so that they come true.

Don't be discouraged by temporary defeat. Everyone faces it, and you need to rise above struggle to get what you want. The things I went through never stopped this book from being created. Likewise, Thomas Edison had hundreds of failures before he got what he was creating. They were just temporary defeats, which led to his invention of the lightbulb.

The next step is to set your intentions behind what you want by creating a fun, loving plan to get it, hustling your plan despite setbacks. Again, align yourself with likeminded individuals who share your goal, and together create a plan to get what you want. Keep plugging away at your plan until you turn your dreams into reality.

This is the spiritual and fundamental framework for accomplishing any dream you aim for and attracting the things you want in your life. There are other techniques, such as vision boards, but the information here is enough to get you started until you read the books listed at the end of this one. You will believe in yourself and achieve your dreams as I did mine, even if it takes much devoted affirming and work to get you there.

God has given everyone an eternal higher self that harnesses the power you need to do or accomplish your dreams with Him, as your co-creator and leader. In other words, God resides in you and leads you, and the power to do anything in His will is there. Through your spiritual growth, you can empower yourself by using positive affirmations and meditations, and you will become unstoppable at positive thinking for yourself and the world!

Sleeping Beauty

During this timeframe in my spiritual advancement, I was personally in need of help for a sleeping problem. Since I was overwhelmed by it, I decided to hand my life over to God. Suddenly miracles occurred everywhere! Timing and success miracles came about in abundance! Angels and ascended masters came out of the woodwork offering me help. One in particular was Jesus. I received many angel numbers indicating the masters were with me. During one particular moment, I was wondering about my sleeping issue when I felt something near me, and a golden cross slowly began to appear floating in my line of vision. I intuitively knew from the way this happened that Jesus was indicating that he was working with me on the issue.

In the days to come, Jesus took it upon himself to teach me how to get the greatest reward before I return to Heaven. He said the best heavenly reward would come if I helped poverty-stricken Africans. Many Africans go through a tougher time with even less than we do. Because of his guidance, I envision myself creating a situation in my future that would raise money for Africa.

The next chapter is about my experience with a very psychic friend and the events that followed in our spiritual online community. Again, it was truly a peaceful place, where psychics could go to share their spiritual experiences and not be judged by anyone. There were so many people who had amazing psychic gifts and were supported by the other members.

Within this online community, I met a very gentle and kind man named Leo Shelton. He shared his gift to communicate with animals, as well as with the spirit realm, through sessions in our spiritual group. I noticed he had a very tremendous gift when he helped someone find their dog by psychically communicating with it. “Animals have unlimited souls, as we do. There are ways we can psychically connect to an animal’s soul to communicate with and help them,” said Leo.

As Leo meditated with a photograph of the animal, he connected to the dog’s energy. Through Leo’s meditation, he received emotions from the animal’s higher self that indicated to Leo the reason the dog ventured anyway from its owner. He also received a very detailed visualization as to its whereabouts. When he communicated these visualizations, the client suddenly realized where to find the dog and recovered him exactly to according to Leo's description.

The client wrote Leo a heartfelt review on Leo's *ChannelingErikMediums.com* webpage. Although everyone has psychic abilities. Leo was born with the ability to connect to animals early in his childhood, and later realized that society's thoughtforms were not correct when they indicated to him that his psychic experiences were only his childhood imagination.

At this point in Leo's career, he wanted to work on his mediumship by offering free or reduced price psychic readings online, some of which were posted live. Leo's consistent ability to speak about a person's most pressing needs were remarkable. These sessions were for people who were random members of our group, whom he didn't know much about. Even though he could have looked up names of family members, and known their individual situations and needs, my perception was that something far more than prior research or an endless winning streak of lucky guesses was going on.

The Good Life

Feeling inspired to hear from Frank Sinatra, I asked Leo to bring him psychically through for a channeled reading. As Leo meditated, I listened to my Frank Sinatra Pandora station to compare the messages I received through my music with Leo's meditation messages. Leo and I were on our computers typing to each other, on a thread in the spiritual community.

As we began, I was wondering if Mr. Sinatra would read my mind and give me responses trough Leo, or if Frank would want me to ask him questions. Miraculously, Mr. Sinatra came through in Leo's meditation, with his distinctive voice, and said right away to Leo, "I want you [Eddie] to ask me questions, son."

Sinatra was reading my mind and answering my question before I asked them to Leo. I explained that I wanted Ol' Blue Eyes to give me advice for my DJ career, give me inspiration, and inform me of any roadblocks to big success.

Mr. Sinatra responded vocally in Leo's meditation, and

this is what Leo typed as the response:

> You are doing pretty good son, you are blessed, and talented. This is what you are supposed to be doing, but be careful who you partner with and contract with. The music/club/entertainment field can be a seedy and negative field, so always stay connected to your higher self/intuition and they will discern [the acceptance of a DJ gig] for and with you. You will feel it in your heart and soul when a gig is right and a blessing for you, and you will also hear and feel it when it's not. If you start having an internal dialog asking questions about the gig, and you feel in your body nervous, or something is not right . . . follow thru on it . . . OR [SINATRA LAUGHS] if you want to test your intuition/higher self, and not follow on their guidance, and do the gig, do it . . . and watch what happens . . . and this will be a learning gauge, because the next time you question,

> or feel something is not right . . . you will know because now you know how it feels in your body.

I believe Sinatra was describing the way I was learning how my soul communicated with me. If I felt nervousness or lower vibes in my body, I already knew that it was my soul communicating with me that something was not right in the situation. I then told Leo that I wanted to meditate and digest that.

Sinatra continued: "Stay focused—you have people around you, who are negative and will try to get you off track with negativity and drama . . . you know this already, don't you?"

I said, "Yes, but it's good for me to hear this."

Sinatra responded,

"Sure . . . meditate and digest take your time, and then go from there. You asked me, so I answered." Sinatra laughed.

Then Leo reported Sinatra coming through visually during the meditation, with a cigar, sitting back in the chair in front of his desk in Leo's formal meditation space. In perfect timing with this, a song miraculously dropped on my Sinatra Pandora station about smoking stogies. I believe that's how the Divine communicates through music. There *are* no coincidences at this level of synchronicity.

I then explained on the post to Leo that Sinatra was DJ'ing for me the entire time Leo's channeling was taking place. Sinatra said to Leo that he likes how I can connect the dots in regards to what Frank is trying to tell me through the lyrics of the songs he was playing. I began to feel that the next song Sinatra played for me indicated big success or fame for me, but the message in the music seemed to be so mysterious that I wasn't sure if I was understanding it correctly. Sinatra then distinctly said, "I want to know your next question, 'Mr. DJ Eddie.'"

I typed back to Leo that I was getting a mysterious message about fame, but I wasn't sure if I was interpreting the music correctly. Leo wrote, "He [Sinatra] immediately lets out a laugh, and he sits there with the cigar in his mouth, legs crossed . . ." Leo felt Sinatra was gesturing, as if to say, "Really, is DJ Eddie asking me this question?"

(After all, God had already answered it.) Leo then

heard,

> Yes, DJ Eddie, there is fame in your future . . . but like I mentioned earlier son . . . BE CAREFUL of who you work/deal/make business/contracts with . . . because it can go wrong in a second, and then you are left wondering . . . what the hell just happened? Stay connected to your intuition/higher self, DJ Eddie.

I told Leo that I really liked to hear that because it was a while since God told me I'd be famous, and I did like the reassurance or confirmation through another's psychic's encounter. During the next song, I actually started getting a message through the music that Sinatra was only wanting me to pay attention to the messages coming through in *his* [Sinatra's] voice [when I channeled him from music in the future]. Then Leo reported, without knowing I was thinking this: Sinatra nodded his head toward Eddie. Leo then reported Sinatra saying,

"Pay attention to my speaking voice, because I will be with you, son. I will help you out . . . and it will be in MY VOICE, so you know it's me."

I knew in my heart that my music channelings were

true; however, I was floored to experience that the messages I was receiving through music were not just nonsense, as I consistently received direct confirmation through another psychic who didn't know specifically what I was channeling on my end. Sinatra then asked for my last question, so I jokingly asked him if he had any new music coming out. He said, "I am inspiring many people at this moment, some know or get a feeling it's me, some don't, but all are inspired, so through this [DJ'ing messages from the spirit realm], in a way . . . I am still putting new music out."

Leo noted that Sinatra took his cigar out of his mouth and tipped it toward me, and just as that happened a very different type of song came on my Pandora, in perfect timing, as if Sinatra were DJ'ing and making a different type of music speak through stations like this. The "different" sounding song was "Shake Señora," by Harry Belafonte.

"I am a music/vocal spirit guide to many," Sinatra said. "Tell Eddie I enjoyed this, and I'm looking forward to helping him out, as long as he wants my help . . ." He then sent Leo an image in which Sinatra's arm was a wing, with me nestled underneath it. This image resonated with me because I felt that he was showing me protection from the negative forces in the music business.

Please re-note that the psychics I know, as well as any psychic in this book have *never* worshiped any of the spirits or angels that came through during psychic meditations or encounters.

In the days to come, I felt so much more confident in my ability to receive spiritual messages through music. God and the angels have spoken to me many times through music. In some cases, it has been through songs, which I have saved for the movie version of this book.

My Near Future

I also intuitively felt drawn to John Lennon one night. I started to see potential future troubles with my career, and I thought, in that moment, that John Lennon would be the perfect one to counsel me about my future fame, so I tuned in my John Lennon Pandora station, mentally requested his messages for me, and channeled it through the music.

(Play "Good to Be King," by Tom Petty.)

John basically said that I would have to get used to my fame. He said that people would make comments about me without really knowing much about me or the person I really am. He said I would have to let it go. He told me to focus on love. He said that my fame could have a strain on my love life. He said that there are higher and lower aspects to fame. During this counseling, I remembered a message I previously received from God during a dream, where God said: "Be simple, be happy."

I felt, in this moment, that it was time to rise above poverty because I feel the need to serve a positive cause on this planet. But I realized I can still be simple and famous at the same time.

When I DJ, I want to be known for DJ'ing for joy, love, and peace. Many will understand it. God sent me many signs that I will be called a king and saint, and receive brotherly and sisterly love from many of those I inspire and help. I never understood the whole saint thing, but I guess I will have to wait and see.

I am setting myself apart as a DJ by playing positive tunes for the sake of the law of attraction. I will say ahead of time, again, that few songs are completely pure or positive. The idea is to just think positively and have loving energy and awareness that all good things are an inward journey, first. If a song talks about getting high, I will be thinking about getting spiritually high, or in other words, spiritually positive. It's about what we want music to mean, not about the jadedness of metaphorical meanings.

I did feel the need to create fame for myself for the sake of the people of the world, so I can make the contribution I want to make. Hopefully, I will be loved in return. I also realize, as an awakened being, that I came to this planet to serve this purpose and my spiritual books and my ideas at the end of this book are going to be part of my positive world contribution before I die.

(Play "Imagine" by John Lennon.)

As I was thinking all this I switched my iHeart Internet radio site to the Calvin Harris station, and I felt the angels when they immediately played, "Feel So Close," by Calvin Harris as the first song. It was clear to me that I would be doing the right thing by making these contributions. I began wondering if the angels thought it would be okay for me to design angel wings on the back of my DJ T-shirts (not because I'm saying I'm an angel, but to spread the message of the angels' light and love).

That very night I politely asked the realm of protection angels to protect me, and then lit some incense to help them chase any darkness away. As I was falling asleep, I saw an amazing image of a very large, soft, fluffy angel looking over my back as I was sleeping. The angel traced wings on my back.

I slept like a baby, and when I woke up, I realized the angel was symbolizing that it was okay to put the wings on the back of my shirt. So, the next day I opened my computer and designed a T-shirt with angel wings.

Soon thereafter, I was sitting on my bed wondering if I would become an ascended master in my time, and I felt Jesus's presence slowly come near me again. I saw half a golden cross floating in front of me. I felt that Jesus was symbolizing I was halfway there. I smiled to myself and as I began to continue working on this book.

I have always had an insatiable desire to master my lifetime, as I looked up to other masters for their ways. I will continue to work at my life and know I've become a master when Jesus shows me his full cross to indicate I've made it. I also received another counseling about my future from the Divine: I turned on my Pandora and "Won't Back Down" by Tom Petty came on right away. I paid no mind to it, and turned it off after a few songs. I then spent part of my day reflecting on my life. It wondered a little about critics, so after watching some very interesting educational videos on Adobe graphic-design software products, I clicked through my browser tabs and the Pandora started playing on its own this time. The divine message hit me undeniably clearly. It played "I Won't Back Down," again! The message was that I should not back down about my spiritual experiences because of people who might have negative opinions about them based on the thoughtforms of traditional American society. I was also reassured by God that people I help would say good things, too.

After this realization, the impact of the message made me walk away to go make a sandwich. When I came back to the computer, the lyrics of the next Led Zeppelin song were saying something, in perfect timing, to the effect that "many men can [will] see the open road." In other words, there will be people who understand what I am experiencing and it will pave the way for a spiritual experience or evolution for them.

I walked away again to continue eating and came back. The next song was "Rock'n Me," by the Steve Miller Band. The follow-up message was very obvious to me. They want me to keep rocking as a DJ, traveling, and making Savannah happy, and my reward in Heaven will be there "in my sweet time." I knew in my heart I would have to rise above any injustices or egos and keep making my contributions through the heart, even if a portion of society didn't understand.

The Divine asked me if I was sure I wanted to be famous, because once it happens I can't take it back. I jokingly replied that I'd be suffering in poverty without it, so why not become famous and make a contribution? I felt that my life was designed to catapult me in this direction, out of poverty, so I chose the pathway that would lead to making a bigger benefit to humanity. I asked the Divine if I should try to become famous another way and they said that I'm really not doing anything t-h-a-t low, and I would be able to find refuge in them and Savannah.

I am not putting down others or disparaging entertainers for what they do, I'm honestly recounting what the Divine told me and trying to show interested souls what I have found. I protected names and voiced positive points about some of the characters, as well. The Divine was correct.

I decided to ask if there was anything else the Divine would like to tell me. They said that everything would be okay and they didn't want me to take drugs. I realized I had no reason to take them, knowing my Dad committed suicide from having schizophrenia and taking illegal drugs.

They also said I don't feel I have much to lose since I

have nothing, but I will sometimes wish I had my old simpler life back when things take off. They also indicated that the people who would auto-discredit me would be mainly those who lacked self-evolved, modern spiritual wisdom. As I reflected on this, I recalled a TV channel that showed religious people voicing the word of God they received from Him while praying (a form of channeling), and no one seemed to discredit the show's preachers or guests, since they were religious. They just called it praying instead of channeling.

It seems that many people may already be intuitively channeling, in one form or another, and are not consciously aware of it. This is probably especially true when people are dreaming. Dreams are mysterious, as channeling can be.

As I concluded my channeling, I showed the divine my appreciation for my counseling and went to bed.

After-Words

As I begin to approach my final words, since God has made me psychically aware that I will be propositioned to have this book made into a movie by a high-level movie producer, naturally there were some details I am leaving out to give the movie a little something that is not in the book.

However, while writing this book on the train to work, mainly for the first three days I literally saw the light of 25 to 50 angels each day. They encouraged me to write what I was thinking in the moment. It cracked me up so many times, because the angels were so joyfully enthusiastic, even about things of very little importance. They even appeared to confirm the thought that they were being silly. I knew from how many angels were around me that writing this book was the start of something big!

The Spiritual Side of Schizophrenia

"And those who were seen dancing were thought to be insane by those who could not hear the music." –Friedrich Nietzsche

First, I would like to mention that I'm not speaking down about the DSM-5 or the "field" of mental health. This field has made a tremendous amount of therapeutic progress in helping patients with psychiatric diseases. I absolutely credit them for it. I am just speaking from my personal experience, as I was diagnosed in 2007, when the field and the caseworkers were less evolved in their practice.

From my point of view, there are two parts to schizophrenia. There is the spiritual part and a mental handicap part. After I became stabilized and more spiritually advanced, I realized that my bouts with the so-called schizophrenic "hallucinations" had been spiritual visualizations that actually existed in, and were created from the 4th (spiritual) dimension, because the spiritual dimension creates what you think about.

I intuitively know this from my experience, as science has no way, that I'm aware of, to track the origin of these visualizations. Because of these spiritual visualizations, I seemed "delusional," since other, not so psychically advanced people couldn't see them, too.

Because I was also mentally handicapped, I couldn't make sense of these spiritual experiences. The darkness could very well give a schizophrenic misinformation, making him sound incredibly abnormal. Because of his handicap, schizophrenics don't understand how off-base they sound when they report the information that they received from the spirit realm.

I needed medication and a concentration on love to limit my vulnerability to demons or darker entities that were telling me to do lower things. I also needed medication to greatly reduce the mental handicap part of the disease that had caused me to be vulnerable to the misinformation or order of the darkness. For schizophrenics, such a vulnerability or mental handicap can result in carrying out persuasive orders from dark spiritual entities, orders we might have dismissed had we been on proper medication. After I was medicated and stabilized, I was able to see that my schizophrenia *is,* actually, partially spiritual. Medication also helps "ground" schizophrenics (there is more on grounding in a later chapter of this book, titled "Healing").

Part of the mental handicap I have referred to, I believe, is also described as the catatonic state, from what I understand of DSM-5. In other words, the mind in this state stops and doesn't process correctly.

Considering this information, schizophrenics aren't as crazy as they usually seem, and it makes sense to me that we are so convinced by our visualizations, because even though they may not contain accurate information, they *are* real experiences. I will describe some schizophrenic episodes to show more specifically what could actually be occurring to patients, based on my experience from the inside out.

This is an extreme scenario: Let's say, for example, a schizophrenic insists dramatically that aliens are shooting at him, but there are obviously no bullet or laser holes in his body. In this case, here are a couple of potential realities that could be causing the schizophrenic to report such an experience.

First, there may be actual demons getting the schizophrenic to believe this is true, either through spiritual visions, voices, or by planting the idea in their mind. However, the mental handicap portion of the disease won't let the schizophrenic understand that he is not actually being shot by aliens in the physical realm. So, in this case, the information is incorrect, but the fact that they have received a message from the spirit realm is real.

In a second paradigm, there may actually be real aliens, creatures, or beings in the spiritual dimension working as in the example above. When the schizophrenic's mental handicap interferes, it prevents him from understanding that this is not actually happening in physical reality, the schizophrenic obviously seems more off base to the non-psychic when reporting such as incident.

Here's another example: An otherwise normally law-abiding citizen has a schizophrenic episode in which "God" commands him or her to shoot people. As you may already understand from my story, this is just a demon posing as God, coercing the schizophrenic to act on lower behaviors. Since the schizophrenic is mentally handicapped, and possibly already afraid of God from religion, the patient obeys the demons out of that fear and starts shooting people.

In the next potential scenario, the schizophrenic is so mentally handicapped that the mind doesn't work enough to know much of what is happening at all, the schizophrenic's mind created a completely false reality of an alien shooting at her, and the information was not channeled from the spirit realm.

I believe the last is a more likely scenario for schizophrenics who are much more deeply handicapped or decompensated. It may one day be found through science that the more mentally handicapped the schizophrenic is, the purer the delusion. However, I think that a report from a schizophrenic who says that there is darkness or light present is more likely to be true than delusional, from my point of view.

I also believe that angels, God, demons, or the ego, as described in Buddhism, can put ideas in an individual's mind. However, I'm basing this on my personal intuition, as science has no way of completely discerning this yet, to my limited knowledge.

I understand that when the spiritual dimension puts ideas in someone's mind, the person receiving this information has no concrete way of knowing if it came from the spiritual dimension or from his own mind. According to a channeled book from the Orin Earth Life Series, when an idea is planted, it feels and seems as if it naturally came from one's own mind. It is up to the experience, knowledge, and sensitive intuition of the person deciphering to figure out where the thought or idea has come from, if at all possible.

Destructive thoughts come from one's ego or from lower entities in the spiritual dimension, and loving thoughts come from higher places such as the higher self or the Divine. Again, a key is to stay focused on God and love, and that will create only God and love in your presence. This should be established as a therapeutic principle for any disease.

The DSM-5's diagnostic criteria state that the schizophrenic is delusional based on "overwhelming evidence." My feeling is that the people who established this criterion were probably not spiritually/metaphysically advanced. Perhaps the diagnostic criteria will be improved when science has a more complete understanding of what is happening in the spiritual dimension.

I believe in the field's desire to heal and help schizophrenics function in society; nonetheless, it was painful in 2007 to have been judged and categorized in a way that defined my spiritual/schizophrenic experiences as delusion, that is, not real. Conversely, this and seemingly most spiritual dilemmas are all in our heads, as they are just a product of what we focus on. Therefore, redirecting concentration to higher, more loving topics is healing in any situation.

However, labeling me as "delusional" did humble me, teach me to be patient and not judgmental to other people's experiences, and for that I appreciate it.

If we find that other patients are experiencing a partially spiritual disease, perhaps we should put the focus on understanding the disease, as well as on a more evolved classification of schizophrenia. After all, our work is always evolving, so one really can't make a concrete diagnosis of schizophrenia until we understand almost everything there is to know about it.

Perhaps there should be studies performed with people

who are advanced spiritually who can help discern what they receive from the 4th dimension, and compare that to what schizophrenics are sensing in their experience. Metaphysically sensitive people might somehow sense things that science cannot yet.

I want to emphasize that the focus must be on helping the understanding with love and healing energy and nothing lower than that. The kind of healing, loving energy we pour into our work will come back to us, and be used to heal others.

I would like the leading clinicians in the world to know that my work on understanding my own schizophrenia is always evolving in the same way their research is. There will be things I may realize after this book is published. I especially invite those who help define the field's diagnosis to contact me if they wish to participate in a group effort to help heal schizophrenics.

I will say in advance that I will decline any studies that would require a change in my medication, as long as I remain stable on the medication I currently take.

After I became spiritual, my schizophrenia began to be healed in many ways. I personally found hope that even though the disease was intense, through positive thinking, I was able to minimize its effects following my second episode, and thereafter.

Therefore, "spiritual health" should be a part of a schizophrenic's recovery. We need to evolve to realize what we imagine in the spirit really becomes true and that we are empowered to think thoughts that *are* higher. Once you become the master of your inner journey, the outer journey will work out, based on the law of attraction and what God is communicating to you.

Looking back on my instability, I feel gratitude for my inner and outer insanity, because it helped me learn life balance! In the long run, any disease can be a gift. To see it this way is empowering and helps you draw on those things you appreciate.

What's the Difference?

Everyone seems to be wondering, what *is* the difference between spiritual awakening and schizophrenia? For me, the main difference is that a person with schizophrenia has a mental handicap that makes that individual become, in spiritual terms, extremely "ungrounded." They are "flying high" and just don't know how to make responsible decisions.

Speaking for myself, being off my medication made me far more ungrounded than I was on it. A non-schizophrenic, psychically sensitive person would probably never experience this level of ungroundedness. I stress that spiritual health should be a part of a schizophrenics' or other behavioral health patients' recovery, because spiritual coping skills are useful for this partially spiritual disease.

Becoming grounded is very important, not just for behavioral-health patients but for those who use the law of attraction, as well as for any individual who wants to have a spiritual awakening. From my point of view, schizophrenics commonly need to become grounded by medication for this to be achieved enough for the schizophrenic to make higher decisions. How to do this is located in the following chapter, titled "Healing."

With regard to the similarities between schizophrenia and spiritual awakening, when I was off my medication, my spiritual experiences were similar to being on medication after I evolved to have psychic ability. However, there were several differences. First, I had many more, and much faster messages while off my medication, and I also experienced more darker entities that gave me incorrect information, or what I believe are lower, lesser forms of truth—based on fear—while off the medicine.

Healing

This chapter discusses the steps that should be taken to help heal the spiritual side of schizophrenia. They could also be a starting point to heal the spiritual side of any disease, or to support anyone who needs to ease their suffering. (Despite this info, you still need to go to check with a doctor and a therapist, as this is not substitute for medication or treatment. This is meant to be just a helpful spiritual beginning.)

A journey to heal yourself begins by loving yourself and putting your healing needs first. Start by relaxing and reflecting on what has a healthy healing effect on you. If you receive an immediate thought about taking drugs or doing anything destructive, these are the thoughts of the ego and you should let them go, because they are not fulfilling in the long run. Focus on guiding your thinking to higher, loving thoughts, and as you go throughout your day, honor the higher part of your being as you peacefully reflect on what is fulfilling to you. Sooner or later you will have a mental list of healing activities you can refer to when you need them.

Meditation can be an excellent start. This can be combined with being immersed in nature to increase the spiritual healing effect. You don't need to push yourself to meditate longer than you feel comfortable. It's also helpful to have a mantra or something positive to repeat in your mind over and over. Mantra repetition can distract you from mental chatter and help you become still and, As Deepak Chopra has explained, if you experience mental chatter, don't fight it. Be at peace with it, and just bring your mind back to repeating your mantra.

A mantra acts like a prayer to the universe. Whatever you're repeating, you are drawing toward yourself, so make sure it is something you want. If you just want to calm down, you can mentally repeat the mantra, "I am calm, God is with me." Take in all the healing energy around you, from nature, God, or your own higher self.

As you become advanced in spiritual healing over time, you won't always need to stop everything just to meditate. Sitting, walking, and eating are all forms of meditation, as long as you enter a peaceful state within.

Another way to heal the soul is by going on a positive self-talk mission. “I can handle anything. I can go to sleep easily. I can heal from anything. I am fearless.” Positive thoughts can actually push you to the next level, spiritually. The more your thoughts are positive, the more they will support your spiritual “comeback.”

Having a healthy spiritual life can help with fears. You can have the protection of God, Jesus, and the realm of protection angels. However, I have found it is has also been effective to simply face my fears. Ask yourself, “What do I have to be afraid of with . . . ?” By putting your fears into perspective, you will find that they dissolve. If you are still afraid after facing your fears, then try to increase your faith. I have found that increasing my faith allowed me to no longer be afraid. Positive thinking, as discussed earlier, will also help you to attract the things you are not afraid of.

For those who believe that spiritual growth is schooling, be aware that God may sometimes do something to take money or resources away for a period of time, so you learn empowerment and increase your faith. But, these are just lessons, and he will make sure everything is okay once you learn what He is teaching you. He reminds me as I type this that He is always with us, even during our toughest times. In summary, I believe that the movement of the planets around the sun every day is proof enough of God's power. We don't die, and there is nothing to ultimately fear. We don't die, we just change form and multiply.

After you develop your healing, self-love, and positive self-talk and work on your fear, you may then need to work on balancing your life. It's beneficial to live with people who have good eating and sleeping regimens. I use meditation, evening rituals, and Reiki to fall asleep. Also, you can ask a licensed psychologist about sleeping hygiene.

I found that it's good to have a hypnotherapist give you your first meditation, because it can build an initial pathway in your mind for calming yourself. Ask a licensed professional about it. Then, as you meditate, you can use the calm pathway that was built during the hypnotherapy session to wind down while the meds kick in (if your psychiatrist has you taking medication). It's also good to start winding down for bed in advance of actually going to sleep, so your heart rate is lower and you are in a calm state of mind before sleep.

Simply eating a lot of fruits and vegetables can boost anyone's well-being. My mental abilities greatly improved when I reduced meat intake and replaced it with a plant-based diet. Again, when you are ready for those steps, being a vegan or vegetarian is said to make you a clearer channel.

If you start to work with angels and invite them into your life from the heart, you could start to see flashes of light, dots, and visualizations that I personally believe are not schizophrenic hallucinations, because they are experienced by many evolved spiritual communities of people who don't have schizophrenia. Don't be afraid of your spiritual visualizations. I believe Angels appear as small dots because they don't want to seem intimidating. They also always come from very high love, like God.

Grounding is essential for awakening, and this is true not only for schizophrenics. I believe it can spiritually help other behavioral health patients as well.

For many spiritual people who discover how to raise their vibration through meditation and stay in the higher energies, the bigger goal is to keep a high vibration while simultaneously staying grounded. I haven't studied grounding techniques deeply, but since the spirit realm works with one's imagination, I have personally developed a way that works for me.

The way that I intuitively ground myself is first to set my intention to "come back down to Earth." The next thing I do was taught to me by a shaman, an evolved American Indian healer whom I will call Raphael. He told me, "Picture two golden rods coming out of your body and connecting you down to the Earth." I find this visualization to be very effective.

These rods can intuitively feel like they are weighting you back down to the planet.

Other people, who resonate with earthier techniques, picture their legs as tree trunks and imagine their feet deeply rooting into the core of the Earth. Some picture the trunks attaching to the bottom of their spine.

It helps to know that we have a silver cord that runs from the bottom of our spine to the Earth, which connects us to the planet in the spirit realm. Using visual techniques—such as envisioning this silver cord in the center of your imaginary golden rods or tree trunks—can also help with grounding.

Healing Continued: Families with Schizophrenia

(Play, "Landslide" (Live) by Stevie Nicks, because it's about the uncertainty of overcoming your life's obstacles.)

When the song describes seeing your reflection in the landslide, I imagine looking in the mirror to see how much I have grown, despite my schizophrenic tribulations. This song was the inspiration for the artwork on the cover of this book.

When I was hit with schizophrenia the first time, it happened so fast that I had no clue what was happening or why I was hospitalized. I just trusted my family.

If you have a family member suffering from schizophrenia, please assure that person that everything is going to be okay. I didn't hear that the first time, because everyone was so worried about how my schizophrenia was affecting others in the family. At that point, my family wasn't talking me through the illness, which would have been the most important support for me to have at that time. Family's must rapidly heal themselves and find the inner strength to stand by the side of their schizophrenic teammate with loving support.

If you are going through a mental illness, there is always light at the other side, no matter how low the illness is. We are surrounded by angels and heavenly beings that many people don't yet see or know how to notice.

According to Michael, my brother, who is also a substance-abuse counselor, "A study showed that a large percentage of people who were considering suicide eventually found that it would have been a bad decision, because their lives became better after they healed from their crisis."

The same was true for my life—I found a huge light at the end of the tunnel. Suffering crises isn't permanent; the more people believe they can grow or live joyfully, the less suffering will be attracted to them.

Schizophrenics who have the capacity to realize they are in need of help must focus on their recovery and give it energy. I spent years researching the wisdom of happiness. Suffering a crisis should be viewed as an opportunity to seek such spiritual wisdom—this is true for schizophrenics, families, and even those who don't have an illness. Any setback in life can be viewed as an opportunity to empower yourself to heal, learn, and overcome, and thus experience your own magnificence or inner God.

Many people were taught by society that a setback is "bad," and therefore, as though on autopilot, we automatically feel "bad" every time there is a setback. But just as we can choose to evolve, we can also consciously choose the way we feel about something. Instead of feeling bad, withhold value judgments, see a setback as an opportunity, and choose to feel good about it. Sometimes happiness is simply a matter of choosing to be happy.

Give everyone the good news on your loved one's progress! A collective family consciousness can attract the circumstances that create positivity for their loved ones—*and the world.*

Your loved one's vibration may need to be raised to help them attract positive things. Although you can't *make* someone raise their vibration, exposing them to something they find to be peaceful, loving, and/or joyful, as well as educating them about their energy, can inspire them to begin to seek it on their own. If you want to sense your loved one's vibration, opening your heart can allow you to receive their energy after a moment or so.

We all need to heal on a daily basis. Some of my most healing moments came simply from being near children or loved ones, nature, exercising, music, cooking a healthy diet, and natural meditation.

Simply guiding your loved one to think of happy things, such as a beach, at the end of a day can take one out of the negativity they were previously focusing on. There are a million healthy paths to helping your loved ones—your intuition is probably already guiding you toward them. Self-love is the first spiritual step in assisting others to heal spiritually.

Psychics, Science, and Schizophrenia

On the topic of psychics, some may eventually bring up the fact that psychics have not always been legitimate or correct. I say, "Yes, but please don't automatically discredit all psychics based on an assumption or the stereotypes associated with palm readers." There have been fraudulent palm readers. I also remind people that when psychics see what lies ahead, they usually claim to be receiving only probable futures and underscore that the future can depend on one's thoughts, and as those thoughts change, so can the future.

Also, please understand the universe can be mysterious. I believe that could explain why some psychics have been right consistently but also wrong a few times. Although psychics make contact with divine beings, perhaps the divine beings can't or don't wish to take 100 percent of the mystery out of life. Because of uncertainty and fear, people want firm answers and concrete evidence, but even science has been wrong, misleading, or mysterious at times.

Guidance is available from the spirit realm for people

who want to evolve. However, many of our answers about how to proceed with something come from the peace, love, and wisdom within ourselves. Speaking for myself, divine beings generally encourage me to use my own judgment and sense things. (See the chapter "Everyone can Channel or Get Divine Guidance.")

Also, becoming psychic should be mainly about getting divine love and guidance, not gaining some kind of egoic advantage. Will God make me famous to serve spirit better? Will God create some type of world peace, eventually? I have faith in it and I will choose to believe it before I see it, as the mystery unfolds itself. Sometimes the darkness is there to bring the light.

I have come to the realization that if life did not contain uncertainty, there would be no growth and learning, and you would not discover your own magnificence. Divine master teachers don't take away learning experiences. But the Divine does guide us if we are willing to stand on our own feet and take responsibility for our own decisions.

Therefore, scientists and psychics should put aside egos and work together with good energy to guide willing people out of their darkness. From my viewpoint, we need to refrain from acting like we know everything before arriving at a conclusion, so that we can continue to see a bigger and bigger picture. I also wish we wouldn't auto-discredit each other based on limited information. We need both logic and faith to work together, while being guided by love. The Divine is giving me this message, in a loving way, as I type: "Listen to your mind and follow your heart."

Schizophrenics who want to receive spiritual messages should be stable on their medication, as well as spiritually grounded before they begin to interpret the spiritual messages they are receiving. When I was unmedicated, my messages came in such abundance and so fast I couldn't always interpret them correctly. There were spiritual entities interfering that made it hard to receive reliable information. When I was medicated and stabilized again, I became grounded enough to make sense of it all. If medication was needed for me to make sense and properly interpret the messages from the spiritual dimension, it could be the same way for others, too.

I want to mention to mental health professionals that according to Doreen Virtue, many people who have had spiritual experience were found not to have anything wrong with their ears or eyes. This was mentioned at one point on her website: *www.angeltherapy.com*

As professionals enter or explore the spiritual side of schizophrenia, I guide them not to be afraid of the darkness they may find tormenting their patients. Be loving, as love casts out fear. The unknown isn't as low as we sometimes fear it being.

Finally, there has been an unknowing in the mental health system with regard to spiritual experiences. Psychiatrists have been instructed to sometimes medicate people for visions or voices because they were educated that visions or voices are "signs of insanity." According to my psychologist brother, Michael, "Diagnosis is complicated and may vary among professionals."

However, I hope my work lends awareness that evolved people are not all schizophrenic, and every voice or vision is not schizophrenia or a reason for non-schizophrenic psychics to be medicated or held in a mental institution. Perfectly healthy psychics who have not been medicated have heard and seen things from the spiritual dimension. The reader shouldn't be concerned that spiritual experiences will turn them into a schizophrenic, especially if no one in their blood-family ever had schizophrenia. (Scientists have found specific genetic markers associated with being schizophrenic.)

People everywhere are choosing to evolve right now and discover their psychic sixth sense. One reason I have been so forthcoming in this book is that I want to pave the way for people to talk more openly about mental health and spirituality without being judged so harshly for it by people's egos, mainstream society, the media, or anyone else. No one on Earth currently has every answer. My thought was that if I could break the ice with this book, perhaps some people who are dealing with schizophrenia will feel that they aren't so low after all and begin to share and be received more widely by others, and will experience more acceptance from an expanding, loving community. First, however, we must accept ourselves.

The Media

I hope the media will realize that they should play a role in non-judgment by portraying mental-health experiences in a wider frame, one that includes higher [more loving] as well as lower behaviors. I wish the media would let go of the fear-based mentality that you must persuade people with fear and drama in order to make money on the news.

Whenever I'm about to make a decision and I am given guidance from the Divine, they usually ask, "Okay, what is a higher decision than that?"

Personally, with love as my highest truth, after I think through my divine guidance, I typically end up making a decision that is several courses higher than the one I would have made.

I wish people in the media would consider this before making a decision about what to promote and attract into mass consciousness, because when we as a people are afraid of the world, we are more prone to disaster on a worldly level. Please understand this. Together, we can make a positive contribution by putting healing, loving energy into this type of work. We are discovering our own greatness here. I believe that's why we're on this planet to begin with. Why not make higher, loving decisions?

As our metaphysical spiritual leaders, who have been considered ahead of their time—from channeling loving, healing, divine information—lead society away from the fear and drama of the ego, we will grow into the peace, love, and joy of an evolved, harmonious, fulfilled society. The reward of living from the heart is very great. Based on his love, I look upon Jesus as the richest person who ever lived.

Because of higher love, compassion, and diplomatic understanding, many people are currently breaking down ancient barriers and no longer looking at gay people with judgmental eyes. We should look at all people as our brothers and sisters, including those who are different from us, as we are all connected children and one with God.

When I see someone who looks more schizophrenic than myself, I feel genuine sympathy for their experiences. We all have troubles, we all have beauty, and we all, in some ways need each other. We are all one!

We are all connected and contributing energy to each other on this planet. When we help others with our energy, we help ourselves. What is your energetic contribution? What is your energy like as it reaches other people, plants, or animals? What is your vibe?

As long as you are still alive, you have time to change the road you're on if you feel it could be a higher course of action or a better contribution. Who among you will be the next spiritual healers or leaders of music, innovation, science, or psychology. Manifest a great contribution by putting out more loving/higher forms of energy!

Everyone Can Channel or Get Divine Guidance

I use the term *psychic abilities* to broadly describe the ways someone can connect to the Divine for guidance, as I explain below. By psychic abilities, I am not referring to the ability to predict the future, unless I specifically mention it in the text.

Everyone is born with psychic abilities, or the means to receive God's signs; therefore, *everyone* has the potential to get guidance from Heaven.

Some parents, however, taught their children to shut down their psychic abilities when they were young. They may have told their child that the things they were hearing or seeing were their "imagination" and not to pay attention to it.

In *Opening to Channel,* Orin and DeBen from the fourth dimension said:

> How many of you have been taught to trust your imaginations? There is a widely

held belief that the imagination is not to be trusted and that only what is scientifically real and provable can be relied on. Yet, many of our greatest scientific inventions come from the imagination.

Learn to trust and honor your imagination.

Albert Einstein "made up" the theory of relativity. Then he proved that it was mathematically possible. Thomas Edison "made up" the electric light bulb and the phonograph, seeing them in his mind before he was able to create them. He believed in the picture in his mind so much that he tried hundreds of times to create the lightbulb and kept going even when everyone else told him it could not be done. Everything in your reality first existed as a thought.

Can you comprehend the richness of your imagination? Your imagination can link you with other universes. It can take you

> backward and forward in time. It can link you with higher minds, and create anything it focuses upon.[28]

It's worth remembering what resonates with you or not. You need to focus on the Divine, yet it is important to interpret if it is coming from a dark, destructive force or a positive one. Is the channeling empowering in a positive way or does it leave you feeling uneasy? If it doesn't resonate with you, it could be coming from a darker force and you should disregard it. Although God has invented humor, if you're thinking, *"The Divine would never say that,"* you may be correct.

I've learned that darker forces can attempt to be nice, too. Spiritual forces can try to pose as something better; it takes experience, good sense, and a correct footing in your heart to learn and decipher where such messages come from. It's good to know that we are always more powerful than darker forces. Usually, the worst they can do to us is try to lie or try to trick us.

It has been said that psychic abilities can either be shut

---

[28] Roman and Packer, *Opening to Channel,* p. 181.

down or can blossom depending on how much the person presently believes in them. The same is true the law of attraction. The more you believe in anything the more real it is.

Channeling can also be a broad term that is difficult to define. Traditionally people meditate and channel what they see, hear, or begin to somehow know.

Some people use a pendulum to ask their divine source a yes or no question. You must first determine which swinging direction is a "no" response and which is a "yes." The divine source will swing the pendulum in the "yes" or "no" direction. You'll notice that, through God, anything moving that you focus on can be a pendulum. I have asked God a question while focusing on a branch and gracefully the wind changes and makes it look like it's shaking in a "yes" movement. For some, it's through music, dreams, or the way a bird soars across your vision, in time with your thoughts.

For me, God has been channeled through signs as tangible as the sign on a truck. As I began to channel Him, I received signs at a frequent, yet gentle and loving pace. They were not originally from my psychic senses. Anyone channeling God may find that He is, at times a challenge–while also being mysterious, loving, and somehow undeniably real. If you do channel God, over the years, you may eventually find that He is literally everywhere, all the time, and always was. The question, then, is not whether God speaks, but rather who is truly listening?

Conclusion

I have spoken openly in this book about schizophrenia in hopes people will understand and learn to be less judgmental about mental health and modern spirituality. I hope to inspire positive and innovative talks and discussions on these topics. I also hope science and spirituality can come together, because I believe they are both basically correct in the grander scheme of things, especially with regard to the creation of the world. (I believe that when God created the universe he burst out, as the Big Bang theory describes.)

I have also spoken about how to access God, angels, spirit(s)–everything in the cosmic consciousness–through meditation, because I wanted to reveal to those who choose to evolve how to access God, Jesus, and angels for the purpose of being guided and growing spiritually.

Accessing the Divine can give you the highest wisdom to guide your life toward improvement. Channeling divine guidance is a major secret of the universe that spiritual people refrain from talking openly about because they don't want to be judged for it.

The reader learned that the Divine has access to everything God knows (contained in the cosmic consciousness). As Doreen Virtue has discussed, angels (and the Divine) can send you signs through just about any means, including electronic synchronicity. Some of these media include Pandora, iHeart, potentially some commercials, and even signs from people or nature that are in perfect synchronization with your thoughts.

You discovered in this book ways to protect yourself from the spiritual dimension with light, Archangel Michael, incense, God, and positive thinking. I taught you the basic wisdom of God's law of attraction. You learned to keep your thoughts, speech, and vibration high because of this law. You learned the basics of master teaching and how we are unlimited through our souls, which are continuously connected to God. One important thing you should take with you in your deepest darkest moments is the subconscious programming you can do to stay positive in the thick of it all. Mentally say, *"I am a genius. I can make it through anything."* If the reader can continuously think positively during any major problem, he or she will find their way out of it much more easily.

The reader also learned that love is the highest power in every universe God created. In fact, all of our problems are there to teach us love in new ways. That is advanced spirituality, for to love your way out of your problems may be one of the fastest ways to come out a winner on the other side.

If the reader is one of the many spiritual persons who have made contact with God or the Divine, I encourage them to stand up with me and tell their story. I believe we need to come together to show the rest of the world that people are evolving and there are miracles that await them, especially for those who wish to grow spiritually or master their lifetimes. The Divine also seems to have a superior "technology" to pull something like this off so perfectly.

Upon the completion of this book, God mysteriously asked that I add that the military and religion have conditioned many people to view spiritual matters in a militant or strict way. He did not comment on whether this is a high or low thing, he simply explained to me the general mentality of the masses. and began to lead me to understand that there is more to write.

Last Story

At the time of writing this book, my girlfriend (I'm not saying whether she is Savannah or not.) made a point to me. I would have to get a job to prove I am capable of working and supporting a potential family, should my dreams not come true within the next four years or so of writing this book. My DJ'ing wasn't a full-time job. So, I humbly got a job at Walmart as a cashier part-time, just for her. Then, my computer got temporarily hacked, and I noticed changes to this book that would have made me sound low if I were to publish it that way. The situation was a stressor, because she thought the hacking was all in my head.

One day, I went to the store and God communicated with me through music that I would be in trouble with the "law." He said I was going to be doing things the only way I knew how and just happen to get in trouble. Since *no one* wants trouble with the law, I was a little worried.

God expressed that He wasn't going to let something really low happen to me. Then the message came to me that I would be speeding, and I wondered if I would get a speeding ticket. He told me to "let it be," and I went to bed that night.

The next night arrived. I was driving home from work when my girlfriend and I got into an argument over the phone about the hacker. I felt sick to my stomach, because she didn't take my word as true and wanted proof that it was happening. At this point, things heated up as I sped into my driveway.

I finally gave in and proved what was happening by showing an original writing and comparing it to what the hacker edited it to say. I was so upset, and I felt she should be able to trust me.

She explained how I lit a fire in a kitchen because I thought it was God commanding me to do it, and said she had trouble fully understanding my reality in certain situations. I explained that I was medicated now, and when the kitchen incident occurred I was unmedicated. She apologized for not believing me, and we decided that she needed to heal from the fire incident so she can allow herself to trust me more when I'm taking medicine.

The next morning, God's amazing sense of humor had

me laughing. He explained, through metaphors in a musical story, that I, "shot my woman down with my argument about the hacker, and that now I'm lonely in a prison [of regret]." He explained that I would be traveling a lot and that my girlfriend and I should cherish our time together, because future time would be limited. This situation was a lesson to me and hopefully others as well, for a couple reasons.

I believe that schizophrenics are misunderstood in a certain way. We may do unacceptable things sometimes if we don't take medicine properly, but even when we do take medicine, we are sometimes labeled or judged as if we are still unmedicated or "crazy." There is a big difference in my experience when I'm medicated compared to when I'm not. It is very painful to be viewed or treated as if we schizophrenics are crazy all the time.

Because of assumptions and labeling I *really* hope this book can pave a new path for people who want to experience God directly and won't be judged for it, as if they were doing something wrong, because they are actually doing it to receive divine guidance, love, or God's humor.

The second lesson is that God can speak on general terms through song lyrics. If you channel through lyrics, you should take what you think is God's general point from the song. This will teach people not to hang on every word of a song so heavily when it comes from God. I have found through my experience that interpreting His words through music and signs is more about a mysterious, creative, meditative, gentle, and individualistic understanding of Him, as He speaks to your experience with love.

God speaks through a beautiful bird soaring high through your line of vision, while you are in deep thought about your dreams. Or the beautiful butterfly I saw through the window, exactly as I typed this, searching outside myself for God's validation of His communications.

Sometimes you may get answers that don't truly make sense until the future events come about. If you get a song that you know God sent to you, and its message is positive but doesn't quite fit with the other songs, remember it for later. When the future arrives, you will recall the message and everything will then make sense.

Spiritual people truly believe that there are no

coincidences, that life can teach us through circumstances. Therefore, the content in this book may have come to your awareness for a reason. I recommend you take time in your life to reflect on this and how this knowledge can put you on a higher path. I'm not pushing spirituality on to you, but you may begin to see how to create a better contribution. You may choose to make it happen before you leave Earth, changing form.

Then, when you're ready, set a time and take action. No matter what happens, with the power of positive thinking we will be shining brightly for everyone to see!

Last Story (I Promise This Time)

In writing this book, I meant only to make a contribution of brotherly and sisterly love to the humanity of our entire world, directly from my heart to the reader's. Since we are all connected as brothers and sisters, remembering love is our highest truth. All there is is love. That is the space in which I have written to my readers, for it is my life purpose to do so.

As I reach the light at the end of the tunnel, I have managed to overcome extreme situations and stand in my own greatness. I am a living example that no matter what happens in life, if you find God, the Divine, or love, you can be free to co-create with God to remove the limitations you place on yourself. This can begin to be possible through spiritual growth mastery and the law of attraction.

I wrote this story because I deeply wanted to inspire people, and I can also say with empathy that I've been there, too. The reader may have read through my insanity and darkness, through suffering that could have made any regular person think about suicide and a gentle, unmedicated schizophrenic set a fire in a kitchen. If I can make it through all of those crises and insanity and think positively enough to manifest life balance, along with this book and its greatness, *anyone can!!* That is the beauty and light of this story–you can do what I did, or better!

Author in the Community

Those of us who know the law of attraction and have reached a point of effectiveness with it can use this law to advance world peace. “You may not feel that one person can have that much effect on the overall energy of the planet, and yet one high, healing thought can cancel out 10,000 or more negative ones,”[29] writes Sanaya Roman in *Personal Power through Awareness*. In another book, she writes, “If you exist in a feeling of love—if you can find it in everything you do, transmit it through touch, through your words, eyes, and feelings, you can cancel out with one act of love thousands of acts of a lower nature.”[30]

In this light, I have a plan to move forward with after this book is published. One aspect of that plan is to hold my own festivals to help promote and celebrate a positive inner journey, through my guidance from God, Jesus, and angels. I would like to use these festivals to help Africa.

---

[29] Tiburon, CA: H. J. Kramer 1986, p. 96.
[30] Roman, *Living with Joy*, p. 88.

If we can unite around such a positive cause, we can collectively put great energy back into the world. I now create music sets that have a greater number of higher thoughtforms, so we can collectively manifest the best while we are being "moved."

If the world defined itself as a peaceful one, maintained a peaceful inner journey, and was conscious that we are a connected body of people, no one would want to harm another, because by doing so, they too would feel that harm. If we saw ourselves as connected, the world would reside in peace. To help make this possible, I am raising awareness for an inner journey.

If you're interested and have experience creating positive festivals, I would like to hear from you. You need a desire to benefit the world, be positive, and be great at what you do. My contact information can be found at the end of this book.

Author As a DJ

(Play, "Runnin Down a Dream," by Tom Petty.)

Since putting spirituality into my music later in my career, I have been guided by God to spin more positive music in an effort to promote light. This music is generally older, mainstream, and works a little better with the law of attraction. Although I try my hardest to spin loving, joyful sounds, Archangel Sandalphen originally described me as being "the gangster of love," probably because some of my music can have a slight hip-hop or street attitude to it. I try to DJ for God in a way that society understands. Therefore, currently, if I do spin a lower song, it is so that it may be used to ground the listener, or for a higher purpose.

Again, my music, books, speaking, and community efforts are my gifts and contributions to promote evolution and growth. Since the presence of God exists everywhere there is love, joy, and laughter, why not work to have more of it? I am also a diverse DJ who has been DJing on and off for over twenty years, so I've been around.

I love my cause and invite the reader to join in, because as you learned, even as an audience member, a positive inner journey is contributing to the world in a good way, through the collective consciousness.

If your audience is about the law of attraction and wants more love, light, and joy, then I am the unique DJ for your following. Check out my mix account below. As a final word, if God invented the festival of Passover, we should feel good about celebrating a positive cause all over the world! Let's go!!

Highlighted DJ Reviews

Nate's Review

I had the opportunity to hire DJ Eddie for a 5k run/dance party of 4,000 people. DJ Eddie was very professional, arrived early, and fulfilled all requests. with this being an all-ages event. DJ Eddie did a great job of playing appropriate music for the occasion. Great mixes, great control, and great execution. We will definitely be using him for future events. Thanks DJ Eddie!

Deslyn's Review

My family and I would like to thank DJ Eddie for an amazing party. His professionalism and energy truly rock the house. Everyone was in astonishment with his outstanding balance and understanding of music. We highly recommend him for any events. . . .

Tony's Review

From the start, Eddie arrived early like I had asked that

he do. He came prepared with his own equipment and extras of everything, which was above what I had asked. In this business, extra is always better. You never know when a needle will break or headphones break, etc. Eddie played the first two hours, which at my club is a critical time to pack the dance floor and bar. Eddie was phenomenal! He read the crowd and performed extremely well, catering to the clientele without skipping a beat. Great job! He's definitely a great asset to have at your event!

Tisha's Review

It was such a blessing to have Eddie as our DJ for our daughter's graduation party! From the start till the end, it was handled with such professionalism, while providing great music for all. I must say I was a bit nervous about trying to provide a mix of music to satisfy all my daughter's friends and ours—you know us older adults, lol. However, Eddie came through with his wonderful performance of music, so all age groups could have a great time together. He handled it so great. Thanks Eddie for helping to make my daughter's graduation day so amazing and memorable. We are very grateful. We will certainly call you back again for our next event!! Cheers!!

MixCloud.com/EddieFaggioli

Highly Recommended Media for Spiritual Growth, Well-being, and Success

I recommend spiritual growth books before any book on attracting money because reading them first could facilitate your path to receiving money. If you go straight to reading about how to attract money, I believe your money could take longer to get to you, if you do not know, or understand the spiritual principals involved in handling it.

1. **The Miraculous Relationships Guided 21 Day Meditation Series*, by Deepak Chopra

2. The Earth Life Series Books, by Sanaya Roman, Duane Packer and Orin

3. *Angel Therapy,* by Doreen Virtue

4. *Angel Numbers 101,* by Doreen Virtue

5. T*he Magic Path of Intuition,* by Florence Scovel Shinn

6. *The Seven Spiritual Laws of Success,* by Deepak Chopra

7. Any book that resonates with your connection to your higher self or God.

Bibliography

1. *Schizophrenia.com/szfacts.htm.*

2. *Health.harvard.edu/newsletter_article/mental-illness-and-violence/.*

3. *Mentalillnesspolicy.org/consequences/victimization.html/.*

4. Steven Covey, *The 7 Habits of Highly Effective People* (New York: Simon & Schuster, 1989), p. 247.

5. Doreen Virtue, *Archangels and Ascended Masters: A Guide to Working and Healing with Divinities and Deities* (Carlsbad, CA: Hay House, 2003).

6. See Doreen Virtue, *Angel Therapy: Healing Messages for Every Area of Your Life* (Carlsbad, CA: Hay House, 1997).

8. Virtue, *Angel Therapy.*

9. Virtue, *Angel Therapy.*

10. *www.angel-guide.com/hierarchy-angels.html/.*

11. Virtue, *Angel Therapy*, p. 163.

12. Sanaya Roman, *Spiritual Growth: Being Your*

Higher Self (Tiburon, CA: H. J. Kramer Inc, 1989).

13. Virtue, *Angel Therapy*.

14. Neale Donald Walsch, *Conversations with God: an uncommon dialogue* (New York, NY: G.P. Putnam's Sons, 1995).

15. Walsch, *Conversations with God.*

16. Walsch, *Conversations with God.*

17. Roman and Packer, *Opening to Channel.*

18. Roman and Packer, *Opening to Channel*.

19. Roman, *Living with Joy: Keys to Personal Power and Spiritual Transformation*

(Tiburon, CA: H. J. Kramer, 1986), p. 88.

20. Roman, *Spiritual Growth.*

21. Roman, *Spiritual Growth.*

22. Walsch, *Conversations with God*.

23. Florence Scovel Shinn, *Your Word is Your Wand* (Virginia: Wilder Publications, 2009).

24. Roman, *Living with Joy*.

25. Sanaya Roman and Duane Packer, *Creating Money: Attracting Abundance*

(Tiburon, CA: H. J. Kramer/New World Library, 2007).

26. Florence Scovel Shinn, *The Magic Path of Intuition*

(Carlsbad, California: Hay House, Inc., 2013).

27. Roman, *Spiritual Growth.*

28. Roman and Packer, *Opening to Channel,* p. 181.

29. Tiburon, CA: H. J. Kramer 1986, p. 96.

30. Roman, *Living with Joy*, p. 88.

CPSIA information can be obtained
at www.ICGtesting.com
Printed in the USA
BVHW04s0237191018
530683BV00017B/200/P